FAT BURNING FACTORS™

Lean Lifestyle Program

The Easy System for Permanent Fat Loss

By Mark Sisson
with Andrew Lessman

Published by Ultimate Health Publications

ISBN 0-9648647-2-X

Printed in the United States of America

First Printing, January 1996

CONTENTS

ACKNOWLEDGEMENTS

No book like this comes together without the efforts of many people. Although far more individuals made contributions than are listed here, the following deserve particular acknowledgement: I'd like to thank Rob Maltas for his valuable insights in making this as "reader friendly" as possible; Patty Gallagher for her assistance editing; Patricia Gin and Joel Ibsen for their design of both the cover and the contents; Fred Zarow for his research acumen; Matt Reed for graciously allowing us to use his West Los Angeles gym "Private Exercise" as the site for all the exercise photos; David Goldner for his photographic insights; and personal trainer/model K.C. Winkler for her help in demonstrating the exercises.

IMPORTANT NOTE

The information in this book is not a substitute for the advice of your physician.

This book contains exercises and dietary recommendations which, depending on your age and physical condition, could require a medical evaluation. Of course, consult with your doctor before beginning this or any other fat-loss or exercise program.

Foreword

By Andrew Lessman,
Founder of The Winning Combination, Inc.

Perhaps the most daunting task any of us will undertake in our lifetime is permanent weight loss. Virtually all of us who attempt to lose weight will fail. Nevertheless, Americans will spend tens of billions of dollars on what continues to be a fruitless pursuit. But there is hope, the **FAT BURNING FACTORS** *Lean Lifestyle Program* is a no-nonsense, easy-to-stick-to method for permanent fat loss.

Unlike other programs and products, we don't tell you what you want to hear about weight loss. Instead, we provide you with everything you need to know to undertake a permanent weight-loss program. All you provide is the motivation and inspiration to make a few **small**—*that's right small*—changes in your life. That's all.

The Fat Burning Factors Program began its development over 16 years ago when we created our original Fat Burning Factors formula. However, I refused to market this product until we also completed an effective, fully integrated weight-loss program. Finally, 16 years later, Fat Burning Factors has a home with the Lean Lifestyle Program for Permanent Fat Loss.

But why did I wait this long? Well, unlike other manufacturers, I do not believe it is ethical to sell a stand-alone weight-loss supplement. It is inappropriate for any manufacturer to give the impression that his products are "magic" fat-burning or weight-loss products. There is no such "wonder pill."

Nevertheless, although Fat Burning Factors offers unsurpassed quality and purity, it is still not a stand-alone weight-loss product. It is designed to work best with a fully integrated program of dietary modification, aerobic activity and resistance training. These small lifestyle changes are what insure the greatest benefits and results from any legitimate weight-loss program. Sadly, there are few if any such programs in existence, so I was compelled to create my own. It had to be simple, easy and permanent. In short, it had to be the best and that's why I collaborated with Mark Sisson.

Mark has been training people to increase their fitness and burn off their body fat for almost 16 years. He has written extensively on these and other health issues for *Men's Fitness*, *Triathlete*, *Bicycle Guide* and *Triathlon Times* magazines, plus he has served as the editor of the *Optimum Health* newsletter. Mark is also the author of two acclaimed fitness books, *The Runner's World Triathlon Training Book* and *Training and Racing Biathlons*. From 1978 through 1983 he was a national-class marathoner and triathlete who finished fourth in the ultimate endurance challenge, the Hawaii Ironman Triathlon. From 1989 through 1991, Mark served as the Executive Director of the U.S. Triathlon Federation, which is the national governing body for endurance multi-sport events in America. Currently, Mark is the Chief Operating Officer of The Winning Combination; an Executive Board member of the International Triathlon Union, the international federation for the sport of triathlon; as well as an accomplished author. The Lean Lifestyle Program is Mark's most recent creation and the culmination of all his years of experience in the areas of fitness and nutrition.

I'm proud to assist Mark in the development of this revolutionary fat-loss program. After reading this book, you'll no longer be a disillusioned dieter "yo-yoing" from one product or program to another. For the first time, you will completely understand how weight loss works and the fat-burning rewards that go with it. Moreover, you will no longer be easy prey to the next marketer of a "lose-weight-fast" program because you'll know the truth.

Now remember, nothing of value comes without some small degree of effort. And, the benefits you derive are always directly related to that effort. Best of luck!

Andrew M. Lessman
Malibu, California 1996

Introduction

*What you don't know can
keep you fat.*

It seems that the entire world is obsessed with losing weight.
Not a week goes by without another fad diet making the *New
York Times* Bestseller List or appearing as the main feature on
the nightly news. Americans currently spend over $40 billion
a year on quick weight-loss programs, diet aids, low-cal meals,
spot reduction and countless other
so-called painless ways to lose
weight. Yet, there are two major problems inherent in our universal quest
to reduce. The first is that most programs are designed not to make you
permanently lose weight, but to make
the authors rich quickly by selling
you "quick-fix" fantasies. They know
that no one in their right mind would
stay on a deprivation plan (diet) for
longer than a few weeks. You may
lose weight for the short time you're

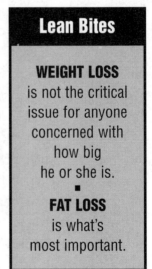

Lean Bites

WEIGHT LOSS
is not the critical
issue for anyone
concerned with
how big
he or she is.
■
FAT LOSS
is what's
most important.

on the diet, but more often than not, you gain it all back (and
then some) as soon as you go off their plan. The second problem is that the information they provide on diet and exercise

is usually outdated by the time it reaches us. It takes years for reliable scientific studies to reach the general public, and, as a result, most "get-thin-quick" publishers are often as much as 10 to 15 years behind the times. Yet exciting new ground-breaking research is continuously being conducted in the areas of fat metabolism, exercise and nutrition. Thanks to the Internet and numerous on-line medical databases, most of this valuable information is available to anyone with a computer, a modem and a little spare time. Knowing this, you might ask why anyone would bother to continue to present outdated information. After all, most of the new research is so much more reliable and compelling. Part of the answer lies in the fact that most people have been conditioned to believe that rapid weight loss can only be achieved through deprivation and dieting (so they look for the latest crazy food combinations) or miracle pills that just melt the fat away. Unfortunately, fat loss doesn't quite work that way.

Perhaps the best example of this "information gap" relates to the very definition of weight loss itself. When you get right to the heart of the matter, weight loss is not the critical issue for anyone concerned with how big he or she is. It has never been the issue—*fat loss* is what's most important. And there is a big difference between the two. You can lose a great deal of weight quickly on a crash diet, but chances are, your short-term loss will consist mostly of water and muscle. This will almost always lead to an even greater weight gain after you go off the diet. The fact is, the best way to lose weight is to lose only your excess body fat while you retain all of your lean muscle mass.

Does that mean it is actually possible to "melt the fat away" as some plans would have you believe? Not exactly, but you can most assuredly train your body to burn its stored fat through a combination of slight alterations in how and when you eat and through your choice of exercise. And therein lies the reason for this book. While many programs focus on one method of losing weight or fat, very few take the time to educate you as to how the body stores and burns fat, and fewer still give you several eating plans and workout options from which to choose. This book will give you the knowledge and the tools necessary to achieve the look and feel you desire, without the daunting prospect of having to give up your favorite foods or having to grunt and groan through a workout program you despise and probably don't believe will work. Obviously, your faith in and your ability to enjoy life on any fat-loss program you choose is absolutely essential to your success.

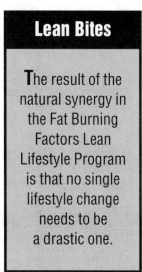

Lean Bites

The result of the natural synergy in the Fat Burning Factors Lean Lifestyle Program is that no single lifestyle change needs to be a drastic one.

Fortunately, the Fat Burning Factors Lean Lifestyle Program will take the guesswork out of what you must do to lose fat. Once you understand the basic information, all you have to do is follow this easy program—step-by-step—and within a few weeks you'll be burning off unwanted fat and exposing a whole new layer of toned muscles underneath. In order to successfully accomplish your fat-loss goal, you will need to understand several straightforward *Key Concepts*, which will assist you in incorporating three relatively easy lifestyle changes: balancing your nutrition, beginning an aerobic exercise program and incorporating some strength training. The elegance of this program is that, while each one of these three simple lifestyle changes has a fat-burning effect all by itself, combined they can have far more than just three times the effect. This multiplying effect is called synergy. Literally, synergy means "the simultaneous action of separate agencies which, together, have greater total effect than the sum of their individual effects."

The result of this natural synergy in the Fat Burning Factors Program is that, by making all three lifestyle changes simultaneously, no single change needs to be a drastic one. For example, by slightly altering what and when you eat, you can change not only how rapidly (or not) you store fat, but also how quickly you burn it. Then, by incorporating a little of the appropriate type and amount of aerobic exercise, you not only train your body to burn more fat while exercising, you can train it to burn more fat while you rest. Finally, by performing just a few simple weight training exercises, you can add more fat-burning potential to your muscles, which will also make the aerobic exercise easier, more fun and the fat-burning effect even greater. All told, three little changes done concurrently will have a surprisingly large fat-burning effect.

NO SACRIFICE NECESSARY

Most traditional weight-loss programs usually involve some

measure of sacrifice. They often require that you give up many of your favorite foods and that you starve and suffer for a few weeks with only a remote possibility that you'll achieve your goal. And even if you make your goal, chances are you won't be willing or able to continue depriving yourself for the rest of your life. Any program that calls for sacrifice is a set-up for failure from the start—and that's not a very effective way to embark on a journey toward any goal. Since in reality no one likes to feel as though they are sacrificing anything in life, most run-of the-mill programs are doomed to failure from the beginning. To avoid this trap, the Fat Burning Factors Program will help you find satisfactory replacements to your current lifestyle, or let you choose from a list of many possibilities, rather than demand that you give up this or do that.

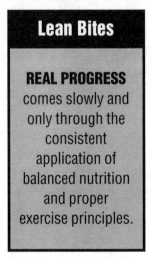

Lean Bites

REAL PROGRESS comes slowly and only through the consistent application of balanced nutrition and proper exercise principles.

Finally, a little bad news: There is no such thing as instant gratification when it comes to fat loss. Real progress comes slowly and only through the consistent application of balanced nutrition and proper exercise principles. Even with the most effective fat-loss program, progress can really only be measured over weeks or months. Noticeable day-to-day changes are unlikely to occur within a reliable program. In fact, certain visible changes can act as early warning signals that you may be doing too much too soon. Such changes are almost always due to loss of water and not fat. The quicker you lose weight on a typical "diet" program, the more likely you are to subsequently rebound with a gain of even more fat. It is almost impossible for your body to burn off more than two or three pounds of fat per week. Therefore, one of the major requirements of a program like the Fat Burning Factors Program is patience. Of course, it's easier to be patient when you can trust that the information you are receiving makes sense. For this reason, unlike other weight and fat-loss programs, the first part of this book is devoted to explaining in easy-to-understand terms how and why you store fat. This knowledge is the key to achieving and maintaining permanent fat loss.

Lean and Mean

What is "lean" and what does it mean?

Our bodies consist of a unique and wonderful collection of cells, tissues, organs and systems comprising things such as muscles, bones, nerves, blood and fat. While many of us might occasionally complain about the aches and pains in our muscles, or about headaches, stomachaches or even broken bones, it's actually our fat that ends up causing us the most grief. Fat is responsible for a multitude of problems from cancer and heart disease to low self-esteem or to simply having to spend extra money on our wardrobe. Unfortunately for most of us, we human beings have a programmed tendency to store body fat. Certainly some of us have a tendency to store fat easier than others, which makes life seem a bit unfair. While the degree to which we store fat may differ among individuals, the mechanisms by which we store and burn fat are the same for each of us. Rest assured, this Fat Burning Factors Program will definitely work for everyone—it just may take a little more or less time for some to see results.

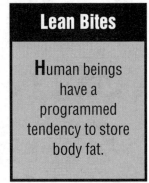

Lean Bites

Human beings have a programmed tendency to store body fat.

All parts of us that are NOT fat are referred to as lean tissue or lean body mass. In general, almost all lean body mass is "active" tissue, which means that in order to maintain itself it must continuously consume energy (calories) throughout the day. Obviously, the largest consumers of caloric energy are the muscles, given the amount of work they are required to do. In addition to the muscles, there are other energy consumers, most notably the brain. However, the brain's use of fuel is insignificant compared to muscle and it can't burn fat. Stored fat, on the other hand, does not consume any energy at all. It just sits around waiting to be used up as a source of energy—or not.

One of the most notable differences between men and women is in how we store and burn fat. Women tend to store fat more rapidly on or near their hips and thighs, whereas men tend to store it more easily around the waist. Although both men and women can train their bodies to burn off fat, for some reason women seem to be a little better suited than men to burning off their fat once they adapt to exercise.

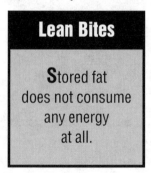

Lean Bites

Stored fat does not consume any energy at all.

What constitutes an acceptable amount of body fat? Much of the answer to that question will depend on your current level of fitness and your goals. Many researchers say that an average ideal body fat level for men is around 15% of your total body weight at age 35; maybe slightly less if you're younger and slightly more as you get older. For women, add 8 or 9 percentage points to account for normal male/female differences, so that if 23% of your total weight at age 35 is fat, you are in a midrange of ideal. Clearly, many people aspire to body fat levels well below the stated average "ideals." Worldclass male athletes are often as low as 5% or 6% or even lower, however, most medical literature shows that anything lower than 5% body fat is borderline unhealthy. Similarly, female athletes often achieve body fat levels as low as 12% or 13%, but in so doing tend to bring about certain health problems such as amenorrhea and anemia. But what about those of us who are not worldclass athletes? The vast majority of us would probably be pleased—and well-served—with a body fat reduction of from 5 to 10 percentage points achieved over a two-month period. While that may not sound like a lot, take a look at an example of how a small change in the percentage of body fat relates to overall weight. A 150-pound woman reducing her body fat from 30% to 23% in 12 weeks, with no loss of muscle tissue, would actually be shedding 14 pounds of pure fat! *Here's how:*

▶ EXAMPLE

At 30% body fat, a 150-pound woman is carrying 45 pounds of fat (150 x 30% = 45). If we know she has 45 pounds of fat, we also know that she has 105 pounds of Lean Body Mass (LBM), because "all of us that is not fat is lean" (150 - 45 = 105 pounds LBM). If she reduces her body fat to 23% and retains her 105 pounds of lean body mass, she will now weigh 136 (105 ÷ by 77% lean body mass = 136 pounds). Thus, in decreasing her body fat from 30% to 23% she will have lost 14 pounds of fat.

Imagine losing the equivalent of 14 pounds of butter or a large Thanksgiving turkey from around your midsection or thighs or under your arms. You might ask whether a 7% decrease in body fat is possible in 12 weeks? It is not only possible, it can be remarkably easy, provided you stick with the plan.

Why be lean?

There are hundreds of good reasons to be lean—but only one good reason to be fat. And that one reason—so we might survive a long period of famine—became unnecessary in this country a few hundred years ago. Not that you need any further prodding to lose those extra pounds, but lets take a quick look at just a few of the benefits that come from a lean lifestyle.

First, holding on to your fat means that your risk for the three largest killers among us will increase several-fold. Many research studies prove that lean people experience far fewer incidences of cancer, heart disease and stroke than even those of us carrying around as little as 20 extra pounds of fat. Fat doesn't necessarily choose to deposit itself just over your gut or thighs. Its negative impact is felt most in your circulatory system, as well as virtually every organ in your body. The physiological changes as a result of this extra fat set the stage for heart attack, stroke, cancer and many other degenerative diseases.

Lean, fit people experience far less lower back pain than obese people. The primary reason is obvious; imagine the strain on your lower back muscles balancing a 10- or 15-pound weight belt hanging off the front of your hips for 24 hours each day. This inactive fat tissue forces your back to work extra hard over time just doing something as simple as maintaining a standing position. When you add activities like playing a little tennis or skiing, you can begin to understand how lower back problems can become major lifestyle compromisers.

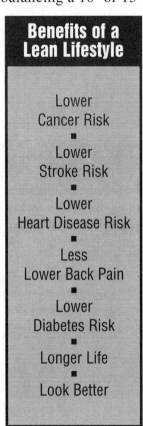

Benefits of a Lean Lifestyle

Lower
Cancer Risk

Lower
Stroke Risk

Lower
Heart Disease Risk

Less
Lower Back Pain

Lower
Diabetes Risk

Longer Life

Look Better

Lean people have lower risk of developing mature-onset or adult-onset diabetes. The primary factor is not exactly that leanness helps to avoid this disease state as much as the fact that fatness tends to bring it about. Several recent studies show that obese people with certain types of diabetes can eliminate, or at least control, their diabetes simply through diet and exercise.

Lean people tend to live longer. While few people embark on a program of diet and/or exercise with the sole purpose of extending their lifespan, it's nice to know that it has been clearly established that one of the benefits of such a program is a longer life.

While living longer is nice, living well is always the best revenge. Lean people not only avoid illness and disease far better than their obese peers, but seem to show an increased enjoyment of life in general.

Last but certainly not least, the main reason most of us choose to lose our fat is vanity. The fact is—for better or worse—the primary motivator for losing fat is so we can look better to ourselves and to others. Even if that is the only reason you've decided to start this program, it's still a very good reason since all of the previously mentioned residual effects are so overwhelmingly positive.

How The Body Works

Whether you like it or not

2

The human body—this basic form that we all share—is the miraculous result of millions of years of evolution. Through countless small genetic mutations and adaptations to the rigors of a hostile environment, our ancestors were able to survive and pass along the very genetic material—the DNA blueprints—that define who we are today. During this long process of survival of the fittest, humans developed many survival skills, among which were the ability to burn some fuels very slowly and efficiently (aerobically) for long treks across the plains; to burn other fuels much more rapidly (anaerobically) when the ability to sprint fast was a life or death issue; and the ability to hunt, scavenge and digest a wide variety of foods which gave us access to these different fuels. Finally, through one of the most useful (and cursed) adaptations of all, our bodies learned to convert any excess food into body fat and to store it around our waist and across our hips for easy transport and future use as fuel during periods of scarcity.

You can imagine that our ancestors must have found this fuel conversion and storage skill a handy adaptation for ensuring our future survival through periods of famine. Thank goodness, or we wouldn't be here without it. Nevertheless, about 10,000 years ago humans must have become tired of the never ending feast and famine routine, because we began to use our brains to produce the kinds of thoughts, reason and logic that allowed us to not only hunt for food more effectively but also to grow and store it. A society based primarily on agriculture emerged and, at least from a survival point-of-view, everything changed dramatically. We no longer had to forage for roots and berries; track animals for days; or wander hungry across the plains for weeks. Most of our food and fuel was now virtually within our reach.

Lean Bites

We can actually train ourselves to burn fat and build muscle using the very same DNA blueprints that would otherwise have us all become plump couch potatoes.

Obviously, we no longer have a need for storing and transporting any surplus fuel on our bodies because our food is essentially available on demand. Unfortunately, our bodies have not yet "caught up" to our minds in terms of evolution, and they (our bodies) still think we must store any excess food as fat in preparation for that long trek across the plains or some period of famine looming in the future. Knowing this, you can begin to see how easy it is for someone to put on 10, 20 or more pounds of fat each year by innocently eating just a few hundred more calories a day than are needed to meet basic energy requirements.

Fortunately, using our same highly evolved brains to analyze and sort through scientific data, we have found that with the right "tools," we can actually train ourselves to burn fat and build muscle using the very same DNA blueprints that would otherwise have us all become plump couch potatoes. You might say that we have learned how to trick the body.

While it might sound slightly devious to think that we might have to trick the body into doing something it doesn't really "want" to do, keep in mind that the body, as a survival-oriented organism, is pre-programmed to conserve energy wherever and whenever possible. If we don't use our muscles they atrophy, which means that they basically shrink both in size and in function. When muscles atrophy, they burn less fuel. This makes sense when you think in terms of the human body as a survival machine bent on conserving energy. But the converse is also true, when you develop and build your muscles, they burn *more* fuel. Certainly, the human ability to respond to hard work (exercise) by building muscle quickly was also a significant part of our survival plan. Otherwise, we might not have had the strength and speed to track and hunt

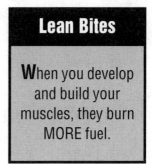

Lean Bites

When you develop and build your muscles, they burn MORE fuel.

for our food. What this means is that while all the unwanted information about storing fat is contained in our DNA, so is all of the useful information about building stronger, leaner muscles and burning stored fat. All we have to do is *choose* which part of that DNA information we want to use and then find ways to encourage the body to use that information.

27

Your choice of how you eat and how you exercise is important because different foods have different effects on your energy levels. Similarly, different exercises (different types of work) cause different adaptations in the muscles. Some exercises promote long, thin muscles that burn higher amounts of fat; other types promote shorter thicker muscles that are able to burn large amounts of carbohydrate quickly, but burn very little fat. The response that a muscle has to a particular type of exercise is very specific and is based on the kind of energy demands that are placed on the muscle. Therefore, if we want to burn fat instead of carbohydrate, we need to choose exercises that cause fat burning adaptations within the muscles. We also need to consume the types of foods that promote the burning of our stored fat. Consider the obvious visible differences between a runner and a heavy-weight bodybuilder: The person who runs 50 miles per week will develop long thin muscles in the legs and very little upper body strength as a response to the specific demands of the exercise chosen. Conversely, someone who just lifts heavy weights will develop large thicker muscles on the upper body and will tend to have more body fat, again as an adaptation to the work done. Yet, even among those people who do similar types of exercise, there may still be noticeable variations based on genetics and the differences in the way they eat. Someone who exercises a great deal and

> ## Lean Bites
>
> **W**e should choose behaviors (eating and exercise) that cause the body to take stored fat and convert it into usable fuel, without cannibalizing muscle.

limits the intake of fats and simple sugars will have lower body fat than someone who does exactly the same types and amount of exercises but increases the intake of fats and simple sugars. This synergy between diet and exercise is undeniable.

Food as Fuel

As you have already discovered, the human body has a basic and primal need for food. Eating food is the only way you are able to derive enough fuel to exist and function as a human being. But just as the engine in your automobile uses different amounts of fuel at different speeds, and gets better mileage with some fuels than with others, virtually the same is true with your body. When we are at rest we use very little fuel. Sleeping, sitting and standing still, for instance, require extremely small amounts of fuel, because your major working muscles— your engine—are not in use. You could say they are "idling." In fact, during these sedentary periods, the largest consumer of fuel is your on-board computer—your brain. Unfortunately, your brain, which doesn't burn that many calories to begin with, is unable to directly access any of your stored fat.

When we "step on the gas" as we do when we walk, run, climb stairs or do continuous heavy labor, our fuel requirements increase dramatically and our "gas mileage" drops. We can satisfy some of this greater demand for fuel directly from the bloodstream in the form of glucose and "free fatty acids" that have been converted from food which we might have eaten a few hours prior. In addition, we can convert some of our stored fuel (fat) into usable fuel to help satisfy this increased demand for energy. Whether or not we take extra fuel out of storage depends on the intensity and the amount of time we spend at these higher work levels. If we're just climbing three sets of stairs to get to the office, chances are that all the fuel requirements can be handled by the glucose nearby in the bloodstream or from the tiny amount sitting right within the muscles. On the other hand, if we ride a stationary bike for 45 minutes, the body will eventually start to take some of its fuel out of both glycogen storage (stored glucose) and fat storage and use it to satisfy the increased demand. This is a good thing. If the ride starts to last longer than, say, 90 minutes, or if we push too hard too soon, we may even start to burn a little muscle tissue as the body seeks other fuel alternatives to make up the difference. This is *not* a good thing. Therefore, the basis of all effective fat loss boils down to this: If we want to lose most or all of our stored fats, we should choose behaviors—*eating and exercise*—that cause the body to take stored fat and convert it into usable fuel, without cannibalizing muscle. That is the "game" of fitness and the path to permanent fat loss. Some ways are better than others, so it helps to know which types of fuel work best with which exercises. Since we'll examine the exercises later, let's discuss fuel (food) first.

There are basically three types of food fuel: carbohydrates, fats and proteins. Each serves a purpose in supplying energy to different parts of the body and at different workloads. Fat burns best at low "speeds" (to continue the automobile analogy) providing nine calories for each gram burned. Fat is potent fuel. Even the most lean among us still has enough stored fat to provide fuel to walk multiple marathons. On the other hand, carbohydrates are most effective supplying energy at higher speeds, and they can do so quite effectively for short periods of time, providing four calories per gram. One minor problem with carbohydrate fuel is that we tend to run out of it easily, so we need to refuel carbohydrates frequently. Lastly, protein doesn't want to be a fuel at all, but does so only during situations that the body thinks are dire emergencies, reluctantly supplying four calories per gram.

▶ Carbohydrates

Carbohydrates provide the most readily available and most easily burned source of fuel for the human body. The terms sugars, starches, digestible fibers, simple and complex carbohydrates all relate to usable forms of carbohydrate. Indigestible fibers, both soluble and insoluble, are also important forms of carbohydrate as they help speed food through our digestive tract. However, we aren't able to derive calories from them because our bodies don't contain the enzymes necessary to break them down.

Some carbohydrate foods such as cakes, candies, fruits, soft drinks and sweeteners contain short carbohydrate molecules that are easily broken down in the digestive tract and become available almost immediately for use by the brain or the muscles. These are generally referred to as "simple sugars." Other carbohydrate foods, such as most vegetables, grains and pastas have longer chains of carbohydrate sugars (often called complex carbohydrates) that take longer to break down, and hence, can act as sort of "time-release" fuels. It is this family of complex carbohydrates that should form the backbone of an energy-rich, low-fat eating program.

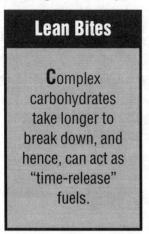

Lean Bites

Complex carbohydrates take longer to break down, and hence, can act as "time-release" fuels.

Regardless of the type of carbohydrate in our food, all carbohydrates are eventually broken down or converted into a usable form of "sugar" called glucose. This high-octane fuel circulates throughout the body in our bloodstream providing short-range fuel for quick bursts of energy. Any glucose molecules that are not used immediately as muscle- or brain-fuel can also be stored in the liver as glycogen or, much to our chagrin, they can eventually be converted into fat. For anyone seeking to maximize his or her use of stored fat, the most important thing to remember about carbohydrate is: *Your carbohydrate consumption will help determine whether you burn your fat off or whether you store more of it.* There is a very delicate balance which, if maintained, will result in high energy and yet very little fat storage. The key is to find that balance. Too much carbohydrate at once, especially simple sugars, and the excess carbohydrate will easily get stored as fat; too little carbohydrate and you won't have enough energy to efficiently burn the fat you have stored. It is a well-established fact that you must have carbohydrate present in order to help burn off the stored fat. In much the same way that the slow-burning logs in your fireplace don't burn well without kindling, without sufficient carbohydrate—whether as "blood glucose" or glucose stored in the form of glycogen—your body is unable to burn fat efficiently. The best strategy requires that you figure out exactly how much of this carbohydrate "kindling" you need to fuel your muscles, but without eating so much that you give the body a chance to convert the "leftovers" into fat. The best way to ensure this is to eat primarily complex carbohydrates along with a little protein, and to spread smaller meals evenly throughout the day. How to do this will be discussed in the next chapter.

▶ Protein

Protein has often—somewhat inaccurately—been called muscle fuel. The truth is, the 22 amino acid building blocks in protein are used primarily not for fuel but to form the structural components of muscle. In fact, the amino acids in protein are used to build and repair most dynamic body systems—including all the enzymes necessary for fat metabolism! Without adequate protein our muscles could not repair and grow from the exercises we do, nor could they even keep up with day-to-day maintenance. But this primary growth function has little to do with protein being used as a source of fuel. Protein only becomes a fuel source under periods of emergency fuel demands when the body is unable to access enough carbohydrate or fat. The best example of this occurs under conditions of extreme starvation. In a typical scenario, when no food has been consumed for 12 to 24 hours the body quickly depletes stored glycogen and glucose. At that point the body goes into "economy mode" in order to save fuel. It actually begins to tear down its own muscle tissue in order to "steal" amino acids from the protein structure of this muscle to send them to the liver to be converted into glucose. This happens automatically. It is a pre-programmed survival mechanism and there is nothing you can do to prevent it (except, of course, to start eating). Since the brain, your body's most vital organ, can only be fueled by glucose, this elegant survival tool kills two birds with one stone. It deals with the starvation scenario by cutting the "fuel overhead" and getting rid of fuel burning muscle tissue and then using that same tissue as brain fuel. The final irony is that our fat stores tend to be spared under these starvation conditions. Of course, in the 20th century, this muscle-cannibalizing survival adaptation has no practical use. Yet, this is exactly what happens when we embark on low-calorie diets, fasting and other drastic means to shed weight; we not only tear down the muscle tissue that allows us to exercise, burn fat, and look toned and is our main source of calorie burning, but we *spare and conserve* the very fat we are trying to burn by not eating. This simple fact is the reason why most traditional "diets" don't work.

> ### Lean Bites
>
> **W**hen we diet, we SPARE the very fat we think we should be burning up by not eating.

The bottom line on protein is that we should regard it more as a growth and maintenance food than as an actual fuel food. Then, provided we have enough quality complex carbohydrates in our diet, we can be confident knowing that our quality carbohydrate and stored fat are providing us the necessary energy, while our protein is primarily being used for growth and repair, and is not being wasted as emergency fuel. Finally, since excess protein can be converted into fat, we should also refrain from taking in too much protein. As you can see, there's a fine line between taking in too little protein and taking in too much. The next chapter will help you determine exactly what's right for you.

▶ Fat

Although it seems to be the bane of everyone's existence, fat still serves a very vital purpose. You might say we can't live with it and we can't live without it. Whenever we are at rest and under some conditions of very low energy expenditure, stored fat provides an efficient and almost unlimited source of fuel. As long as some carbohydrate is present (whether as blood glucose or as stored muscle glycogen or liver glycogen), fat will continue to provide a substantial portion of basic maintenance fuel. That's how we are designed.

For example, if your body needs to burn 1200 calories every 24 hours to maintain itself without any activity, chances are that up to 80% of that energy (almost 1000 calories) will come from burning fat. Some of that 80% will come from your stored fat and some of it will be from the fats you ate today that have not yet been stored but are still circulating as triglycerides and "free fatty acids" in your bloodstream.

If you are one of those lucky individuals with a "high metabolism" or a "fast metabolism" your body may require twice as many calories as the rest of us just to keep you functioning at rest. Many athletes who train an hour or more a day experience this luxury. They actually burn off twice as much fat as non-athletes while just resting! This is largely due to the fact that these people—regardless of their size—have more active muscle tissue, which requires a constant supply of energy all the time.

Lean Bites

There's no magic to what an athlete does to train his or her body to burn fat—it's a matter of the adaptations that occur from doing aerobic exercise with a little strength training.

The ability to burn fat effectively at rest is just one way in which athletes are able to maintain low body fat levels. The other method involves the ability to use higher amounts of fats while exercising at relatively high intensities. This not only allows them to access a nearly unlimited supply of stored fat, it also delays the eventual depletion of smaller carbohydrate reserves. Since carbohydrate depletion ultimately causes performance to drop, this ability to burn fat translates into better endurance. Still, there's no real magic to what an athlete does to train his or her body to burn fat—it's just a matter of the adaptations that occur from doing aerobic exercise in conjunction with a little strength training. Luckily, the same principles apply to you seeking to burn off all your fat. The next few chapters will explain how you can easily teach your body to do exactly the same thing.

Step 1: Eating Right

Reduce the fat you store by adjusting the way you eat

In the previous chapter we proved why the typical diet doesn't work. We demonstrated why each of us needs a certain number of calories every day to avoid having our body go into "economy mode" by becoming too efficient and actually cannibalizing itself. Low-cal diets are literally a waste of energy. But there are some secrets to eating that can actually enable your body to burn off more of your stored fat and to store less fat to begin with. In order to learn how those secrets apply to each of us individually, it will be

The Key Fuel Concepts

▶ Know your weight and your body fat.
▶ Know the amount of "fuel" that's just right for you.
▶ Don't starve—eating too little can be worse than eating too much.
▶ Never eat a large meal close to bedtime.
▶ Graze—don't gorge.
▶ Eat foods you enjoy—don't feel as if you are sacrificing anything.
▶ Learn to read and understand food labels.
▶ Make complex carbohydrates the mainstay of your diet.
▶ Drink plenty of water.
▶ Be certain you get all necessary vitamins and minerals.
▶ Avoid being misled by the term "low-fat."

necessary to get a more detailed picture of who you are and exactly what your unique fuel requirements are. If you learn to apply these *Key Concepts*, you'll be on your way to a low-fat, high-energy lifestyle.

KEY CONCEPT 1 *Know your weight and your body fat.*

Knowing your weight is a breeze. Everyone has a scale nearby—sometimes *too* nearby! As long as you weigh yourself at the same time of day—and no more than twice a week—you can get a reasonably accurate picture of your true weight. Knowing your body fat percentage is slightly more complicated, but it is what will help you determine how much of you is lean body mass and, therefore, how much fat weight you can "afford" to lose.

There are several different ways to measure body fat, all of which are painless. The most accurate way—but also the most expensive—is a process known as hydrostatic weighing. In this case, a technician actually weighs you in a tank of water and calculates your "fat weight" by applying a mathematical formula based on the fact that fat floats. Basically, the more you float or the less you weigh under water, the more fat you have. Another popular fat-testing technique, called near infrared or NIR, involves placing a small beam of infrared light on the biceps muscle of your arm and having a light sensor record the amount of light that is dispersed by the fat in your arm. Since fat tends to distribute itself proportionately throughout the body, the more fat you have on and in the muscles of your arm, the more fat you probably have elsewhere. NIR is also the main method our USDA presently uses to grade fat levels in the meat we buy in the supermarkets. Yet another method, referred to as bioimpedence testing, measures the resistance of your body to a very tiny—and painless—electrical current passed through you by a special device. "Resistance" can be defined as the inability of an object to conduct electricity. As fat is a great resistor of electricity, the higher the electrical resistance measured by the machine, the higher your body fat.

After all is said and done, perhaps the easiest and least expensive method of determining your body fat is with body fat calipers. By simply pinching some of your subcutaneous (beneath the skin) fat just above your hip bone, you can measure to within a few percentage points exactly how much body fat you have distributed over your body. The beauty of testing body fat with calipers is that you can make the measurements in the privacy of your own home and you can measure as frequently as you like. Fat caliper testing is also the least expensive, since all of the other methods require that someone like a physician or a health technician perform the measurement using expensive equipment.

Regardless of the method you choose to determine your body fat percentage, keep in mind that whenever you measure again—to compare before, during, and after—you should use the same method. The reason for this is because even though the accuracy of one method over another may differ, the relative change in your body fat will be consistently demonstrated accurately if you measure by the same method each time.

Now, it's time to measure your body fat and determine a few baseline numbers which will help you plan what and how much you should eat.

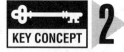

KEY CONCEPT 2 ***Know the amount of fuel that's right for you.***

You will recall from earlier discussions that only lean tissue consumes fuel; fat tissue does not. Also, if we know how much of you is fat, we can easily determine how much of you is lean and, therefore, the total weight of you that is comprised of fuel-burning tissue. It is this figure, also called Lean Body Mass, that we can use to calculate the total amount of calories you need each day and the amounts of each of the different fuels (fat, carbohydrate and protein) that are right for you. Therefore, once you have arrived at a body fat percentage number (from one of the methods in *Key Concept 1* above), you simply plug it into the equation below to arrive at your total fat weight:

▶ *CALCULATE YOUR FAT WEIGHT*

Weight _____ lbs

✖ % body fat _____

Fat Weight _____ lbs

Then subtract your fat weight from your total weight to get your lean body mass:

▶ **FIND YOUR LEAN BODY MASS**

> Total body
> weight _____ lbs
>
> ▬ Fat weight _____ lbs
>
> **Lean
> Body Mass _____ lbs**

Now to find the total number of calories required by your body to keep you energized throughout a moderately active day and still require you to burn some of your stored fat, multiply your LBM times 14. The figure you arrive at will be the number of total calories necessary for you to maintain your lean body mass while you burn away body fat.

▶ **DETERMINE YOUR DAILY CALORIES**

> Lean
> Body Mass _____ lbs
>
> ✖ ___*14*___
>
> **Daily Calories
> Required _____**

There's one final calculation. In order to get the ideal break-down of fats, protein and carbohydrates, you'll want to refer to the chart on the next pages in order to break your caloric figure down into the different fuel components:

41

DAILY CALORIES AND GRAMS

▶ *Based On Your Lean Body Mass*

LBM	Calories	Carbohydrates		Fats		Proteins	
+/- 3lbs	Total	Calories	(Grams)	Calories	(Grams)	Calories	(Grams)
80	1120	616	(154)	280	(31)	224	(56)
85	1190	652	(163)	297	(33)	240	(60)
90	1260	692	(173)	315	(35)	252	(63)
95	1330	728	(182)	333	(37)	268	(67)
100	1400	768	(192)	351	(39)	280	(70)
105	1470	808	(202)	369	(41)	292	(73)
110	1540	844	(211)	387	(43)	308	(77)
115	1610	884	(221)	405	(45)	320	(80)
120	1680	928	(232)	414	(46)	336	(84)
125	1750	960	(240)	441	(49)	348	(87)
130	1820	1004	(251)	450	(50)	364	(91)
135	1890	1040	(260)	473	(53)	376	(94)
140	1960	1084	(271)	490	(54)	392	(98)

LBM	Calories	Carbohydrates		Fats		Proteins	
+/- 3lbs	Total	Calories	(Grams)	Calories	(Grams)	Calories	(Grams)
145	2030	1116	(279)	508	(57)	404	(101)
150	2100	1160	(290)	522	(58)	420	(105)
155	2170	1200	(300)	540	(60)	432	(108)
160	2240	1240	(310)	560	(62)	456	(114)
165	2310	1274	(319)	576	(64)	460	(115)
170	2380	1310	(328)	594	(66)	476	(119)
175	2450	1350	(338)	612	(68)	488	(122)
180	2520	1386	(347)	630	(70)	504	(126)
185	2590	1422	(356)	648	(72)	520	(130)
190	2660	1462	(366)	666	(74)	532	(133)
195	2730	1500	(375)	684	(76)	546	(136)
200	2800	1538	(385)	702	(78)	560	(140)
205	2870	1578	(395)	720	(80)	572	(143)
210	2940	1618	(405)	734	(82)	588	(147)
215	3010	1658	(415)	752	(84)	600	(150)

EXAMPLE

Phil has determined he has 157 pounds of Lean Body Mass. In order to calculate the amount of fuel he should take in daily, he refers to the chart on pages 42-43. Rounding to the nearest five-pound increment, he sees that at 155 pounds of LBM, he should take in a total of 2170 calories each day. To assist him in planning his meals, the chart also tells him how many calories and grams of each fuel constitute the total caloric value. As a result, he reads across the line and sees that it will take 300 grams of carbohydrate to supply the 1200 calories that will come from that fuel; 60 grams of fat to provide another 540 calories and 108 grams of protein to equal 432 calories from protein.

▶ *Or, as a more general rule of thumb, multiply your total calorie allotment by the following percentages:*

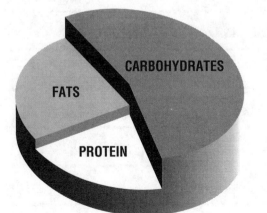

Carbohydrates
55% - 65 %
▼
Fats
20% - 25%
▼
Protein
15% - 20%

Now you know exactly how many total calories are required by you in the Fat Burning Factors Program as well as what portion of that total should be in the form of carbohydrates, fats and protein. To get the weight in grams of each fuel, refer to the numbers in parentheses on the chart or just divide protein and carbohydrate calories each by four and fat calories by nine.

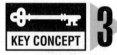

3 *Don't Starve. Eating too little can be worse than eating too much.*

Remember the example we used earlier in which a starvation diet caused the body to go into "economy mode" and consume its own precious muscle tissue? Obviously, that is exactly the situation we want to avoid. Therefore, it is important that, *each and every day*, you consume the amounts of protein, fat and carbohydrate food you figured in *Key Concept 2*. There is no extra credit in the Fat Burning Factors Program for eating less than the amount required to maintain lean body mass. In fact, you'd be hindering your progress by skimping on your eating. Of course, on the other hand, anytime you exceed those fuel numbers, you postpone the opportunity to burn stored fat. Therefore, your best results will come when you try to stick closely to the plan. There's a foolproof method in *Key Concept 5*.

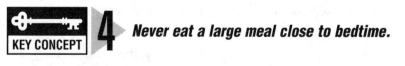

4 *Never eat a large meal close to bedtime.*

Most people the world over—not just Americans—seem to use the evening meal as a reward for a long day's work or as a social reason to consume large amounts of food and drink. This may be effective as a means of gathering together to rejoice in the successes of the day, but it represents complete sabotage for anyone seeking to burn off stored fat. The only thing a large evening meal does is encourage your body to store *more* fat. Especially if you've "sacrificed" by not eating much food earlier in the day. Think about it. Late in the day, after your work and workout is finished, you fill yourself up with calorie after calorie of a "well-deserved" multicourse meal. It sounds enticing, but a few hours later you head off to sleep and all your body does for the next several hours is convert almost all of that food into stored fat. Perhaps, if you're lucky, you might get away with a hundred or so grams of carbohydrate being diverted to the muscles and liver to replace the glycogen you burned in a workout (provided you did your workout), but the rest of the carbohydrate, most of the protein and all of the fat will just get sent to storage while you sleep. Can you imagine a more devastating setback to a fat-burning program?

If you can pace your food intake over the day, you'll find you won't be so hungry when the evening meal rolls around. And even if you find you are especially hungry, there are several choices you can make among foods that will give you a satisfied sensation of fullness without the likelihood of these foods

> ## Lean Bites
>
> **If** you can pace your food intake over the day, you'll find you won't be so hungry when the evening meal rolls around.

being converted to fat while you sleep. A large plate of steamed vegetables or a large salad with a vinaigrette dressing are just two examples of such a meal.

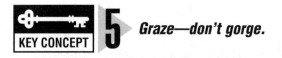 *Graze—don't gorge.*

Many of us have the unproductive habit of gorging on one or two large meals each day. A typical pattern of skipping breakfast (short-term starvation) and then having a huge lunch or dinner to compensate, leaves us at the effect of wide mood swings due to radical changes in our blood sugar levels. Skipping breakfast also encourages the cannibalization of our precious muscle just as we're starting out our day. Finally, to make matters worse, it prompts the storing of even more fat later on in the day when we eat more than we should. Under this pattern,

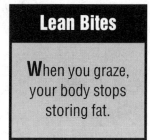

Lean Bites

When you graze, your body stops storing fat.

the reason we tend to overeat later in the day is because our brain gets chemical messages from the bloodstream that tells the brain we are *starving*, so the brain then instructs us (through our appetite) to eat as much as we can get our hands on. Then, to make matters worse, the brain tells the body to store as much as it can as fat—a double whammy! One of the easiest ways to avoid this vicious cycle; to ward off this hunger; to maintain an even level of energy all day; and to ensure that you don't consume your precious muscle tissue is to "graze" throughout the day.

The idea behind grazing is to divide your food up into three, four, even five, smaller meals and spread these out over the full day, rather than having one or two large meals. This habit of grazing takes a little thought and planning ahead of time, but it's easy to adopt. First, plan on a substantial start to your day (i.e. more than just a cup of coffee!) by having a breakfast that contains at least a little protein and a significant amount of complex carbohydrates. See the sample breakfast menus in Chapter 6. Balance out your energy level midmorning with a small healthy snack, such as a cup of yogurt and a piece of fruit, or an energy bar. Then have a light sensible lunch, another small midafternoon snack and a small evening meal. The total calories you consume during the day will be manageable and your feeling of energy will be higher than ever. See pages 54 and 55 for an explanation of how this works.

> ## Lean Bites
>
> The idea behind grazing is to divide your food up into smaller meals and spread these out over the full day.

There is yet another benefit that comes from grazing. When you provide yourself small nutritious high-energy meals throughout the day, your body begins to adapt to what it senses as a continuous supply of energy. Since your body operates under the principle of energy conservation and "use it or lose it," this continuous supply of food helps your body decide that it doesn't need to store any more fat and therefore reduces its production of the enzymes that are required to store fat. When we have fewer of these fat storing enzymes, we aren't able to store as much fat, even if we want to. This fact alone should make grazing worth a little extra effort.

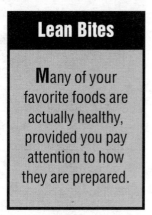

KEY CONCEPT

6 ▶ *Eat foods you enjoy.*

Many people have the incorrect notion that a healthy eating plan, by definition, can only consist of small quantities of bland, unappealing foods. Nothing could be further from the truth; yet, this has been the "diet" industry standard over the past few decades. While there are certainly healthy foods that aren't necessarily appetizing and a large number of great-tasting foods that are very unhealthy—and should probably be avoided when possible—there is also a vast array of healthy foods that are great-tasting and provide plenty

Lean Bites

Many of your favorite foods are actually healthy, provided you pay attention to how they are prepared.

of choices and variety to anyone interested in staying on a healthy eating plan. As you will see from the list of meal plans and snack foods in Chapter 6, many of your favorite foods are actually healthy provided you pay attention to how they are prepared and to the portion or serving size. There is no law in the Fat Burning Factors Program that states you must suffer through unappealing meals. On the contrary, by giving you many such choices, we think you'll be much more inclined to stick with the plan and, as a result, achieve the results you desire.

KEY CONCEPT

7 ▶ *Learn to read and understand food labels.*

A generation ago, most people had no idea what sorts of ingredients could be found in the foods they were eating, much less the exact amount of each nutrient per serving. Today's new food labels, which are called Nutrition Facts, make smart eating almost fool-

Nutrition Facts

Serving Size 1 Entree
Servings Per Container 1

Amount Per Serving

Calories 280   Calories from Fat 110

	% Daily Value*
Total Fat 12g	18%
Saturated Fat 5g	25%
Cholesterol 40mg	13%
Sodium 610mg	25%
Total Carbohydrate 27g	9%
Dietary Fiber 4g	16%
Sugars 5g	
Protein 16g	

Vitamin A 45%	•	Vitamin C 2%
Calcium 10%	•	Iron 20%

*Percent Daily Values are based on a 2000 calorie diet. Your daily values may be higher or lower depending on your calorie needs:

	Calories:	2000	2500
Total Fat	Less Than	65g	80g
Saturated Fat	Less Than	20g	25g
Cholesterol	Less Than	300mg	300mg
Sodium	Less Than	2400mg	2400mg
Total Carbohydrate		300g	375g
Dietary Fiber		25g	30g

proof. If you learn to understand and follow the label, you can't go wrong. There are a few basic elements to a food label that require a little explanation:

Be aware that everything on the food label will be relative to the serving size printed on that label. Not that you need to restrict yourself to the serving size specified, but be aware that when you double the serving size, you also double the amount of each nutrient and calorie in that serving.

The right-hand column contains the percentages of Daily Values of each of the nutrients listed. As your label clearly states below, these percentages are based on a 2000 calorie per day diet in which 30% of all calories are from fat. These daily value numbers are meaningless if your total calories per day are more or less than 2000 and if you stick to a diet of 25% of calories from fat. The grams listed in the column on the left are far more meaningful.

Total Calories and Calories from Fat are the first numbers you'll read on the label that have real meaning. From these you can determine the percentage of this food or this ingredient that comes from fat. Simply divide fat calories by total calories to get that percentage number. As a rule of thumb, you should try to stay away from anything that derives more than one-third of its calories from fat.

The next major category is Total Carbohydrate. While this number gives you an idea of overall carbohydrate content, the more interesting numbers appear just below it. The higher the Dietary Fiber, the better and the lower the Sugars the better (since the remaining balance is likely to be the more desirable complex carbohydrate).

Next is Protein, expressed in grams. Try to keep a tab throughout the day of the total grams of protein you're consuming. A little protein with every meal helps even out energy levels by reducing the amount of insulin you produce as a response to the carbohydrate content of your meals.

Make Complex Carbohydrates Your Primary Fuel.

Knowing that you'll want to limit your total fat intake to 70 or fewer grams per day, and that it doesn't take much protein to fill out the quota of 60-100 grams per day (depending on your lean body mass), all that remains to sort out is the types and amount of carbohydrate you should eat. All carbohydrate foods are made up of varying length chains of one or more simple sugars (e.g. glucose, fructose, galactose, lactose, maltose, etc.). Ultimately, however, all carbohydrate forms must be broken down by the gut and the liver and converted to glucose or stored as glycogen before they can be used for energy.

Additionally, our bodies have yet another built-in survival mechanism to ensure we don't just waste any excess of the carbohydrate we eat. When too much glucose enters the bloodstream all at once, our bodies respond by secreting the hormone insulin, whose primary function is to "sop up" all this excess glucose and store it in our cells as glycogen or, eventually, fat. The problem caused by eating a very high carbohydrate meal and dumping a large quantity of simple sugars (very short sugar chains) into the bloodstream is that the body often overreacts and puts more insulin than is needed into the bloodstream. The result is that more glucose is taken out of the bloodstream than was present even before the simple sugar was consumed. The net effect on us when this happens is that we store more fat and start to feel lethargic and listless. This is because the brain, which is highly dependent upon circulating glucose to function properly, is suddenly robbed of its only fuel by virtue of the automatic insulin effect. When we eat a high carbohydrate meal we get an immediate sugar "rush" as the food starts to break down and a great deal of glucose is released. Shortly afterward, a surge of insulin causes all that glucose fuel to be removed from the bloodstream and we suddenly feel weak, sluggish, unable to focus and certainly without the energy to begin a workout. It usually requires another meal or snack to raise our blood-sugar levels to normal again (see pages 54 and 55). Therefore, it serves us best to select mostly the complex carbohy-drate foods that allow for the slower, steady release of glucose into the blood-stream, rather than those that cause a quick, short-lived rush of glucose, fol-lowed by an insulin crash.

Lean Bites

Select mostly the carbohydrate foods that allow for the slower, steady release of glucose into the bloodstream, rather than those that cause a quick, short-lived rush of glucose, followed by an insulin crash.

If you have ever wondered why your energy levels are different throughout the day, and why you are hungry even though you eat large meals, perhaps it's related to the types of food you eat and when you eat them. The two graphs on the following pages compare what hap-pens to our energy levels and fat storage on a standard diet (page 54) against the energy levels and enhanced fat burning that occur when we graze (page 55).

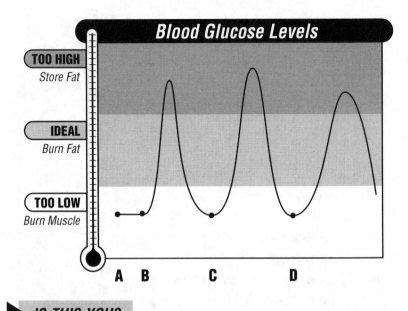

IS THIS YOU?   When you wake up (A), your blood sugar is low primarily because you haven't eaten for 10 or 12 hours. A quick cup of coffee and a sugar doughnut (B) might give you a quick burst of energy, but that is soon followed by a drop in blood glucose to below the ideal range. You wait until noon or even later to eat lunch (C) but by then you're so hungry you eat more than you should, so once again your blood glucose rises too high. Your body responds by producing insulin to "sop" it all up, even storing it as fat. As a result your blood glucose drops too low and by 3 p.m. you feel lethargic and sleepy. Carrying this low blood sugar into evening, your brain signals you to eat a large dinner (D), which then sits in your gut all night being converted to fat while you sleep. Your day has been punctuated by wide energy and mood swings, you've stored even more fat and you've possibly cannibalized some precious fat-burning muscle.

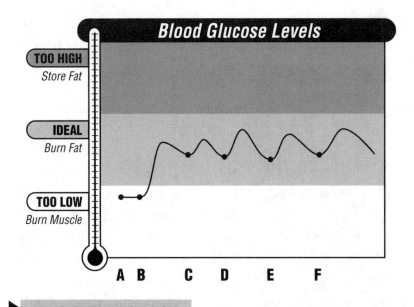

THIS SHOULD BE YOU When you awaken (A), you eat a sensible breakfast consisting of complex carbohydrates and a little protein (B). Your blood glucose will rise into the ideal range. Midmorning, as the energy effects of your breakfast begin to subside, you have a healthy snack (C) which prevents your blood glucose from dropping below ideal. Again, around midday, a small lunch (D) consisting of a mix of complex carbohydrates, protein and a little fat boosts your energy, but not so much that you store any excess as fat. A light healthy mid- or late-afternoon snack (E) accomplishes the same thing and by dinnertime, all you need or want is a light supper (F). The result: Your energy levels have remained even all day, your appetite has stayed low, you have burned more fat, you have stored less fat and you haven't burned up any precious muscle tissue.

One of the easiest ways to identify foods that provide a slow, steady supply of glucose without an energy crash is to refer to the "glycemic index" of each food. The glycemic index, or GI, was developed as a means of measuring how quickly different foods were converted from their various carbohydrate forms into glucose once inside the digestive system. Foods with the highest GI convert to glucose the fastest, pure glucose having a GI equal to 100. Notice that even some "starchy" complex carbohydrate foods, such as potatoes can have a fairly high GI.

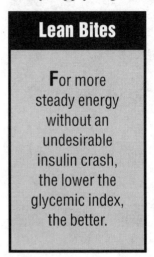

Lean Bites

For more steady energy without an undesirable insulin crash, the lower the glycemic index, the better.

Some other foods, such as lentils, often considered more of a protein food than a carbohydrate, actually have lower, more favorable GIs. In fact, adding a little protein to a high GI food can have a similar moderating effect.

A high GI doesn't necessarily mean that a food is bad, nor does a low GI mean a food is good. For instance, high GI foods often stimulate faster energy replenishment via glycogen replacement than low GI foods when eaten immediately after strenuous exercise. This is desirable in some instances. Low GI foods seem to enhance performance slightly more than high GI foods when eaten a few hours before a workout. *The general rule of thumb is that for more steady energy without an undesirable insulin (sugar) crash, the lower the glycemic index, the better.*

GLYCEMIC INDEX CHART

▶ BREAKFAST CEREALS
All Bran 42
Corn Flakes 84
Cream of Wheat
    (Instant) 74
Grapenuts 67
Rice Chex 89
Rice Crispies 82
Shredded wheat 67
Special K 54
Total 76

▶ CRACKERS
Rice cakes 82
Rye crispbread..............63

▶ DAIRY
Low fat yogurt
    (sweetened) 33
Ice Cream 30
Whole milk...................27
Skim milk 32

▶ FRUITS
Apples 36
Apple juice 41

Apricots (dried) 31
Bananas 53
Cherries 22
Grapefruit.....................25
Grapefruit juice 48
Grapes 43
Oranges 43
Orange juice 57
Peaches (fresh) 28
Pears.............................36
Pineapples 66
Plums 24
Raisins..........................64
Watermelon 72

▶ LEGUMES
Baked beans 48
Black-eyed beans 42
Butter beans..................31
Chickpeas.....................33
Green beans...................30
Lentils 29
Split peas (yellow)........32

▶ PASTA
Fettuccini......................32

GLYCEMIC INDEX CHART

▶ PASTA
Linguine 46
Macaroni 45
Spaghetti 41
Rice pasta 92

▶ RICE
White, long grain..........50
Brown............................55
Uncle Ben's
    converted................38

▶ STARCHES
Bran Muffins 60
Blueberry Muffins........59
Carrot Muffins..............62
Waffles 76
Bagels............................72
Oat bran bread 47
Pumpernickel bread......41
White flour
    wheat bread 70

Whole-meal flour
    wheat bread 69

▶ SWEETS/SNACKS
Honey............................73
Mars Bar.......................68
Nacho chips..................73
Potato chips 54
Peanuts 14
Popcorn 55

▶ VEGETABLES
Carrots...........................71
Corn (sweet)..................55
Potatoes
    Baked 85
    Mashed...................73
    Sweet......................54
    White......................56
Pumpkin 75
Tomato Soup 34
Yams.............................51

Adapted from: Foster-Powel, K. & Brand Miller, J. 1995. International Tables of Glycemic Index. American Journal of Clinical Nutrition 62: 871s-893s.

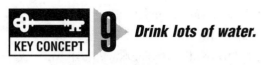 **Drink lots of water.**

Water is the medium through which virtually all biological functions take place. Most of our lean body mass consists of water. We simply can't live without it. It is especially important for anyone attempting to burn off stored fat to consume lots of water. In fact, 10 eight-ounce servings a day is a minimum recommendation. While that might sound like a lot, keep in mind that juices and some soups contain mostly water. Even vegetable meals and salads contain appreciable amounts of water. However, don't count alcoholic or caffeinated beverages within your water consumption group, since these drinks can act as diuretics and cause water to leave the body through the urine. Add another glass or two of water for each of these diuretic drinks you have during the day.

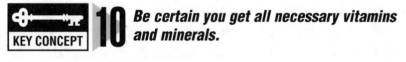 **Be certain you get all necessary vitamins and minerals.**

Just as carbohydrates, fats and protein are all necessary to provide for fuel and repair, there exists a whole group of nutrients, called micronutrients, which are absolutely essential for any and all metabolic processes to take place. They could be called the "spark plugs" that allow our fuels, including all our stored fat, to burn. These micronutrients include vitamins, minerals and other molecular entities. While a well-balanced diet that includes lots of fresh fruits and vegetables will generally also contain adequate amounts of most micronutrients, many of us aren't able to eat sufficiently well on a consistent basis, especially when exercising or watching calories. One of the best ways to be assured you are getting all the necessary fat-burning nutrients is to take a daily supplemental multi-vitamin multi-mineral formula.

KEY CONCEPT 11 *Avoid being misled by the term "fat-free."*

Probably the greatest misconception among people interested in losing fat is that they begin to believe they can eat virtually anything that's fat-free and not have to worry about the results. This is largely due to overzealous advertising campaigns on the part of the food industry to sell their newest fat-free or low-fat foods. Unfortunately, a label claiming "fat-free" simply means that none of the calories in that particular food come from fat. "Fat-free" doesn't mean that the food has been suddenly rendered "healthy" or "low-cal." It often means that the calories that replaced the fat now come from simple sugars (even if artificial sweeteners are used). The danger here, as we learned earlier, is that these simple sugars can cause a quick surge of energy followed by a precipitous drop in energy level as our insulin rushes in to carry the glucose away for safe keeping. Not only do we experience this negative effect as a feeling of fatigue, but these simple sugars can also be converted to fat very easily. Therefore, the net effect in terms of fat storage on our bodies is the same with some "non-fat" foods as it would have been had the food contained its original fat.

There's yet another hidden pitfall: Simple sugars don't give the same sense of satiety or fullness that fats do, so we often tend to eat more of a "fat-free" or "reduced-fat" food than we might have had the food contained the original amount of "satisfying" or "filling" fat. There's nothing wrong with eating more when a non-fat food consists primarily of complex carbohydrate with lots of fiber (fruits and vegetables, for instance), but when we eat "calorie dense" fat-free foods that don't leave us with a feeling of fullness we can often take in three times the calories before we realize we're full. Some researchers now theorize

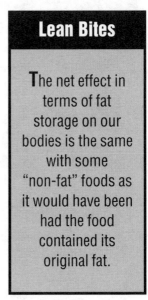

Lean Bites

The net effect in terms of fat storage on our bodies is the same with some "non-fat" foods as it would have been had the food contained its original fat.

that the alarming increase in obesity in this country over the past 10 years may be due to consumers believing that labeling something fat-free means they can eat anything fat-free with abandon. Despite all the hype surrounding fat intake, obesity and health and an increased "awareness" of nutrition and exercise, the average American in 1993 weighed eight pounds more than the average American in 1980. If it's true that people have actually cut back on their fats over the past 10 years, it's also likely they've more than made up for it with an increase in simple sugars. To avoid this predicament, read all labels with a "healthy" skepticism.

Step 2:
Working It Off

*Increase the fat you burn
through aerobic exercise*

Now that we've learned exactly what fuels to eat and when best to eat them, the next step is to begin the process of burning off our excess stored fat through aerobic exercise.

If the medical, health and fitness industries had to pick one panacea—the one perfect cure-all for almost every illness or affliction known to man—aerobic exercise would come the closest. Regular aerobic exercise has been shown to reduce susceptibility to almost all illnesses from the common cold and flu to heart disease and cancer. This is due to the positive physiological changes it causes, including a significant boost to the immune system. Other afflic-

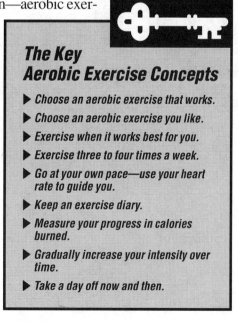

**The Key
Aerobic Exercise Concepts**

▶ *Choose an aerobic exercise that works.*
▶ *Choose an aerobic exercise you like.*
▶ *Exercise when it works best for you.*
▶ *Exercise three to four times a week.*
▶ *Go at your own pace—use your heart rate to guide you.*
▶ *Keep an exercise diary.*
▶ *Measure your progress in calories burned.*
▶ *Gradually increase your intensity over time.*
▶ *Take a day off now and then.*

tions like gout, diabetes, varicose veins, lower back pain and even hemorrhoids can often be prevented simply through doing regular aerobic exercise. Aerobic exercise can increase energy, mental alertness, general productivity and self-esteem while it decreases depression. And of course, aerobic exercise is the single most effective way to lose body fat. Until only recently, with the advent of modern transportation, regular exercise was how we got around; it was the one thing every human had in common. In many ways we were healthier and certainly less fat in those earlier times.

> ## Lean Bites
>
> **A**erobic exercise can increase energy, mental alertness, general productivity and self-esteem while it decreases depression. And of course, aerobic exercise is the single most effective way to lose body fat.

A good session of aerobic exercise can burn off anywhere from a few hundred calories to a few thousand. That alone could be enough motivation for some people to begin a program. But there are those among us who might cringe at the thought of walking two miles just to "equal" the dollop of cream cheese on the bagel we had for breakfast. For those of us who are less inclined to take up exercise for the sake of just burning calories while we work, there is some additional *great* news. Much of the recent research has demonstrated that aerobic exercise actually trains the body to raise its basic metabolic rate *all the time*, even during periods of rest. In other words, after just a few weeks of regular aerobic activity, the body "adapts" by burning more calories at rest in addition to those it burns during a workout. Moreover, an increased number of those calories burned at rest come from fat. At some higher levels of intensity, the body may burn as much as one calorie *extra* at rest for every calorie it burns during exercise. Imagine burning 500 calories during a workout and then burning another 500 (over and above what you'd normally burn) during the next 24 hours by just going through your normal paces. It is theorized that this happens because the

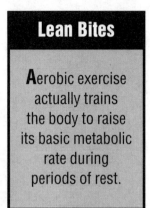

Lean Bites

Aerobic exercise
actually trains
the body to raise
its basic metabolic
rate during
periods of rest.

body begins to adapt to regular exercise by preparing in advance for the next session. Some researchers think that the body may take fat out of storage during recovery and use some of it to provide the extra fuel needed for recovery while depositing some of it directly at the muscle cells where it can be more easily burned during the next session. Finally, there is strong evidence that a regular exercise program trains your body to burn more fat per workout than you normally would burn if you were exercising just once in a while. There's no doubt about it, doing aerobic exercise is one of the best "deals" around when it comes to squandering and eliminating stored fat.

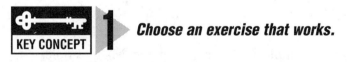

KEY CONCEPT

Choose an exercise that works.

As funny as it may sound, not all forms of aerobic exercise are great at causing our bodies to burn off unwanted fat. Certainly, *anything* you do in the way of exercise will lead to some amount of positive change, but there are certain aerobic activities that simply far outdo others. Running or cross-country skiing rank among the most effective at shedding fat. On the other hand, swimming ranks low. While swimming is a great cardio-vascular exercise (good for the heart and muscles), it is just not as effective at getting rid of fat as running or cross-country skiing. One reason is the fact that, even at temperatures of 80-degrees plus, most pool water is still some 20 or more degrees "colder" than our core body temperature. Because water conducts heat away from the body 200 times faster than air, when we immerse ourselves in this "colder" water, sensors under our skin detect body heat being conducted away and respond by depositing more thermal insulation (fat) underneath the skin and over the muscles. You may correctly point out that Olympic swimmers still look great—and they do—but they actually maintain body fat percentages six to seven percentage points higher than equally well-conditioned runners or cyclists. None of this is to say we shouldn't swim; swimming is still a fairly good calorie-burning exercise and all-around conditioner, just not the best fat burner.

> ## Lean Bites
>
> **N**ot all forms of aerobic exercise are great at causing our bodies to burn off unwanted fat.

Golf is another example. Golf is a great game. Many people spend hours and hours over the years in pursuit of the perfect game, but the fact remains, golf is just not a great calorie burner. If you choose it as your main activity, you should be prepared for less than impressive fat-loss.

So what does constitute a great fat-burning exercise? The best fat-burning exercises involve the continuous repetitive use of any large muscle groups. Walking, running and cycling are all great fat-burners because they require continuous use of many muscles in the thighs, lower legs, and buttocks. Cross-country skiing or using an indoor cross-country ski machine adds the extra calorie-burning benefit of upper body muscle involvement as well as the legs. Rowing machines, ladder-type climbers and the new aerobic "riders" also force you to use both upper and lower muscle groups.

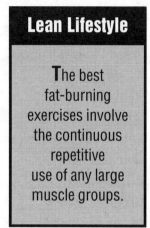

Lean Lifestyle

The best fat-burning exercises involve the continuous repetitive use of any large muscle groups.

The point is, the more muscles you can use during your aerobic activity, the more "demand" you tend to place on your heart to pump fuel into the working muscles. As you'll soon see, your increased heart rate is the best measure of how hard you are working.

Following is a chart of the most popular aerobic activities and approximately how effective each is at burning calories:

CALORIES BURNED PER MINUTE

Exercise	YOUR TOTAL WEIGHT IN POUNDS					
	110	130	150	170	190	210
▶ Basketball	6.9	8.1	9.4	10.6	11.9	13.1
▶ Boxing	11.1	13.1	15.1	17.1	19.1	21.1
▶ Cycling						
leisure; 5.5 mph	3.2	3.8	4.4	4.9	5.5	6.1
leisure; 9.4 mph	5.0	5.9	6.8	7.7	8.6	9.5
racing	8.5	10.0	11.5	13.0	14.5	16.1
▶ Dancing						
aerobic, medium	5.2	6.1	7.0	7.9	8.9	9.8
aerobic, intense	6.7	7.9	9.2	10.4	11.6	12.8
▶ Golf	4.3	5.0	5.8	6.5	7.3	8.1
▶ Hill Climbers	7.0	8.3	9.5	10.8	12.0	13.3
▶ Jumping rope						
80 per min.	8.2	9.7	11.2	12.6	14.1	15.6
125 per min.	8.9	10.4	12.0	13.6	15.2	16.8
145 per min.	9.9	11.6	13.4	15.2	16.9	18.7
▶ Racquetball	8.9	10.5	12.1	13.7	15.3	16.9
▶ Running						
11.5 min. per mile	6.8	8.0	9.2	10.5	11.7	12.9
9 min. per mile	9.7	11.4	13.1	14.9	16.6	18.3
8 min. per mile	10.8	12.5	14.2	16.0	17.7	19.4
7 min. per mile	12.2	13.9	15.6	17.4	19.1	20.8
6 min. per mile	13.9	15.6	17.3	19.1	20.8	22.5
5.5 min. per mile	14.5	17.1	19.7	22.3	24.9	27.5
▶ Skiing, *cross-country*						
level, mod. speed	6.0	7.0	8.1	9.2	10.2	11.3

Exercise	YOUR TOTAL WEIGHT IN POUNDS					
	110	**130**	**150**	**170**	**190**	**210**
▶ **Skiing,** *cross-country*						
level, walking	7.2	8.4	9.7	11.0	12.3	13.6
uphill, max. speed	13.7	16.2	18.6	21.1	23.6	26.0
▶ **Swimming**						
crawl, slow	6.4	7.6	8.7	9.9	11.0	12.2
crawl, fast	7.8	9.2	10.6	12.0	13.4	14.8
▶ **Tennis**	5.5	6.4	7.4	8.4	9.4	10.4

This is how to use the information in the previous chart to calculate the calories you'll burn doing your aerobic exercise:

▶ **EXAMPLE**

Jill weighs a total of 130 pounds. She attends aerobic dance classes at her local health club. The workouts last 45 minutes, after a brief warm-up, and are usually at a medium intensity. Referring to the chart, Jill would see that a 130-pound person burns 6.1 calories per minute doing aerobics at this level. 45 minutes multiplied by 6.1 = 275 calories per workout. The reason she uses her total weight and not just her Lean Body Mass to figure her calories per minute is because she is carrying around all her fat weight as well as her lean weight when she exercises.

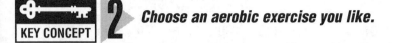

KEY CONCEPT 2

Choose an aerobic exercise you like.

While this might sound obvious, often the temptation for the first-time exerciser is to look at the chart and to pick an exercise based solely on how many calories it burns. The danger in this is that you might pick something that, while a great calorie-burner, you wind up doing less because it's too difficult or too discouraging in the early phases. The key is to pick an exercise (or exercises, because there's no less benefit from doing several different forms) that you enjoy. This way there is a greater likelihood you will do the exercise regularly. Remember, the point is not to suffer, but to alter your lifestyle slightly by incorporating something that is good for you and that you feel good about doing. Perhaps this is why so many people choose walking as their primary aerobic exercise; it's something we all know how to do, it's easy, it's enjoyable (especially when you walk with a partner), it can be done outside or inside equally effectively, and it allows for a variable pace.

> **Lean Bites**
>
> **C**ross-training alleviates the boredom that may come from doing the same type of exercise every day.

Many people choose to alternate between two or more different types of aerobic exercise. This practice, also known as cross-training, accomplishes several goals. First, it alleviates the boredom that may come from doing the same type of exercise every day. Second, it allows for more complete recovery from one type of exercise when you alternate with another type. Finally, most people find it both challenging and rewarding to become proficient at several different aerobic activities.

KEY CONCEPT 3 — *Exercise when it works best for you.*

There is no right or wrong time of day to exercise. In fact, whatever time you select will be the right time for you as long as you know you'll be able to consistently fulfill your commitment to exercise. The main consideration should be to pick a time when you know you will be able to exercise. Many people find that exercising the first thing in the morning is a great way to start off the day. That's usually when there are the least distractions. It's quiet in the early morning, and there's a sense of accomplishment one achieves finishing a workout before doing anything else. In addition, a morning workout not only gets the blood flowing for the remainder of the day, but it also establishes an increased metabolism that encourages fat-burning for the next several hours. One trick to help you follow through on morning workouts: Lay out your workout clothing before you go to bed, put them on as soon as you wake up and don't take them off until you've completed your exercise for the day.

On the other hand, there are those of us who just can't seem to get it together first thing in the morning, or who have other considerations like getting the kids off to school or getting to work on time. Some studies also show that our heart rates, our manual dexterity and our reaction times are not at their best first thing in the morning, but function best later in the day between noon and 9 p.m. For those people, exercising right after work or possibly on a lunch break might work best. The point is, do it when it works best for you.

One of the myths that surrounded aerobic exercise until recently was that you had to do all your aerobic exercise at once; (i.e., you couldn't break up a 30-minute workout into three 10-minute segments or two 15-minute segments without diminishing the benefits). Much to the delight of many time-constrained workout fans, that myth has recently been dispelled. In fact, the research shows that your results can be just as impressive doing three 10-minute walks (or runs or rides or climbs) as doing 30 minutes steady. At last, those of us who claim we can't find 30 or 45 minutes to work out on certain days can find solace in knowing that we can accomplish our workout by taking a 10- or 15-minute break at work to climb stairs a couple of times a day, or by taking a shorter morning walk and then another walk in the afternoon or evening.

KEY CONCEPT **4** *Exercise aerobically 3-5 times a week.*

Since aerobic exercise "teaches" the body to burn stored fat, it is important to keep the lessons coming frequently. Research supports the popular notion that for aerobic exercise to be most effective at burning fat, it must be done at least three times a week. Any less than that and the body isn't given enough of a reason to create better fat-burning systems. Once or twice a week and you may burn actual calories during the workout, but you won't burn as much fat, and the long-term effect of continuing to burn fat throughout the day just won't happen as effectively.

Knowing this, you might think that if three times is good, seven or eight workouts a week must be great. Fortunately in this case, more is better only up to a point. It appears that five aerobic workouts a week is probably optimal, particularly if you are also doing your weight training twice a week in addition. Any more than five and you start to put a little too much stress on your body's recovery systems. Each time you do a fat-burning workout, you want to give the body a little rest period from which to recover and respond by manufacturing a few more fat-burning enzymes. You want the lesson to "sink in," so to speak. For this reason, the Fat Burning Factors Program suggests that you commit to doing at least three aerobic workouts a week, shoot for four or five, but don't do more than five aerobic workouts per week.

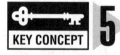

KEY CONCEPT 5

Go at your own pace—use your heart rate to guide you.

The general rule of thumb with aerobic exercise is: The harder you go for any length of time, the more calories you burn. Although any activity you do to boost your workload is preferable to sitting around doing nothing, more is usually better. Therefore, your basic workout goal should be to increase the intensity of your aerobic training from week to week and month to month. However, it makes no sense, nor does it offer any benefit to exercise so hard in the beginning stages that you quit early because you are too tired, or that you go so hard that you are not able to recover from one workout to the next. Luckily, there is a proven formula for "pacing" yourself during workouts that ensures that you stay within that optimal training zone and do neither too little nor too much work. This formula utilizes your heart rate (pulse) as an indicator of just how hard you are working and therefore allows you to go at your own pace.

Lean Bites

The higher the intensity at which you exercise, the more calories you'll burn.

The heart rate training formula works under an assumption that we each have a Maximum Heart Rate at which our heart will beat under the most difficult workload; and that, unless we are worldclass athletes, we almost never want to work out so hard that we reach that heart rate. Instead, we should choose a range of heart rates that works best for each of us individually, based on a fixed percentage of our maximum heart rate. The surest way of learning your own exact maximum heart rate is to have a physician test you on a treadmill while you are hooked up to a special monitor. Short of that, there is also a simple formula most people have used successfully for decades that involves subtracting your age from 220 to arrive at your "theoretical" maximum heart rate in beats per minute. While this 220 minus your age formula may not give you an exact maximum heart rate, a large body of research has demonstrated that it will generally be within a few beats either side of your actual maximum heart rate.

▶ **CALCULATE YOUR MAXIMUM HEART RATE**

220
━━ *Your age* _____

Maximum heart rate _____*bpm*

Now that you have determined your theoretical maximum heart rate, you can arrive at what percentage of that rate you wish to do most of your exercising. For beginners it's best to start at the lower end, which is generally around 65% of maximum. After a few minutes of gradually warming up, most of the time you spend exercising should be at or around 65% of your maximum heart rate.

▶ **EXAMPLE**

Take, as an example, Lois. She is 42 years old and will begin a walking program this week. To figure her maximum heart rate she should take 220 minus 42 (her age) = 178 Beats Per Minute (BPM). Then, to arrive at her best beginning workout pace, she multiplies 178 by 65% and arrives at 117 BPM. For the first several weeks of her program, she will try to keep her heart rate around 117 BPM after a brief warm-up. If her heart rate climbs too much above this number, she can either slow down a little or stop a while. Of course, if she's below 117 BPM, she'll try to pick up the pace a little.

How do you measure your heart rate? Many indoor exercise machines have built-in heart rate monitors (also called pulse meters) which make tracking heart rate a breeze. For people who are gadget freaks or who just want to track and record everything as accurately as possible, there are several popular brands of small portable heart rate monitors worn on the wrist that sell for as little as $80 and are available in most sporting goods stores. Finally, you can easily estimate your heart rate simply by finding your pulse with your middle finger placed over the artery on your neck or wrist. Using a stopwatch, or even a watch with a sweep second hand, count the number of pulses in a six-second period and multiply times 10 (or add a zero) to get the number of beats per minute.

Those who are already advanced aerobic exercisers might elect to work at higher heart rates than the starting suggestion of 65% of maximum. Heart rates as high as 75% or 80% of maximum can be quite comfortable for someone just a few weeks into a fitness program. Remember, while you don't want to poop out early during your workout or jeopardize your recovery by doing *too* much, the higher the intensity at which you exercise, the more calories you'll burn both during and after the workout. The net result will be that your body will take more fat out of storage and use it to fuel all this activity.

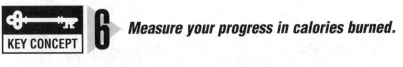

KEY CONCEPT 6 ▶ *Measure your progress in calories burned.*

Some people like to measure the miles they've walked; others count floors climbed and still others just watch the clock. However, the true common denominator among all aerobic activities is that any and all work you do can be measured as "calories burned." Almost every piece of indoor exercise equipment manufactured nowadays has a "calories burned" readout. There are also some easy formulas you can use to figure calories burned without using fancy monitors. The point is that by measuring calories burned, you can compare past workouts with current workouts and you can create similar workloads doing completely different activities. You also get an idea of how much calorie-burning extra credit work you can accomplish by taking the stairs instead of the elevator, by walking

Lean Bites

By measuring calories burned, you can compare past workouts with current workouts and you can create similar workloads doing completely different activities.

to work instead of driving or even by standing and pacing around your home or office while you talk on the phone.

If you use equipment that does not have a calorie counter, or if you exercise outside, there are two primary methods for determining how much calorie-burning you are accomplishing. The first method is to refer back to the activities chart on pages 68-69 to get a sense of what effort level you are working at and multiply the amount of time spent at that level (in minutes) by the number of calories which that exercise burns per minute.

Another way of figuring calories burned when you are running or walking is to use this general rule of thumb: Each mile covered equals 100 calories, regardless of the speed. While this is a little less precise than taking a reading directly from your treadmill or bike console (since the amount of body weight you are carrying will affect the equation a little), it can still provide you with a good relative measure of just how much calorie-burning work you are accomplishing from day to day. Of course, this method also requires that you know the distance you cover in a given workout. For example, if you walk briskly for 4.5 miles, you would multiply the distance (4.5) times 100 (calories per mile) and arrive at an impressive 450 calories burned.

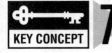 **7** *Gradually increase the intensity.*

When you become aware of the amount of calorie-burning work you are doing in each workout, you can much more accurately and methodically determine your short- and long-range fitness goals. Just as a journey of 1000 miles begins with one step, the simplest way to make regular progress in your fat-burning plan is to burn a few more calories each day. Thus, if you burned 260 during today's workout, shoot for 270 tomorrow and 280 during the next one. After a very short while, you may find yourself routinely burning up to or over 500 calories per workout. Seven days of this (which should take a week and a half if you are exercising aerobically four to five times a week) and you will have burned up 3500 calories, or the equivalent of one pound of body fat. Keep in mind that for each calorie you burn during a workout, you burn another over the next 24 hours. Therefore, the 500 calories you burn during the actual workout results in yet another 500 calories (over and above your normal metabolic rate) being burned during the remainder of the day. The work you do, combined with your new higher resting metabolic rate, combined with your proper fuel (food) consumption throughout the day can

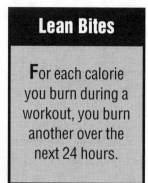

Lean Bites

For each calorie you burn during a workout, you burn another over the next 24 hours.

result in your safely and painlessly losing more than a pound of body fat per week. That's the natural synergistic effect we spoke of earlier.

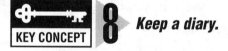

KEY CONCEPT

8 *Keep a diary.*

As reluctant as many of us are to keep accurate records of something as mundane as a daily workout, keeping a logbook record of each workout is a good habit to develop and will accomplish several things. First, it will enable you to monitor your progress from day to day and week to week. Fat loss is not the world's greatest instant gratification pursuit. In order to see how far you've come, you'll want to have a written record. Second, a journal can have a "motivational" effect. If you don't exercise on a day you had intended to, that will also be part of the record. And finally, the minor discipline of spending three or four minutes writing notes about a workout is a subset of the kind of discipline necessary to do your workout each day. The writing reinforces the training and the training reinforces the writing. A sample logbook page appears on page 143 in the back of this book and can be easily copied for repeated use.

KEY CONCEPT **9** *Take a day off now and then.*

As we discussed earlier, our bodies have information in the form of DNA blueprints that allows us to adapt to the positive stresses of exercise. The main adaptations to aerobic exercise include building more lean muscle tissue as a result of greater workload demands and creating a more effective fat-burning engine as a result of increased energy demands. While it is the work we do that creates this positive "stress," it is the rest period in between, as well as a good eating plan, that gives our bodies time and materials to recover, adapt and build. The good news is that a day off now and then is not only allowed in the Fat Burning Factors Program, it's strongly encouraged. A total day off from exercise not only assures that the body has at least one occasional 48-hour period between workouts to completely build, but it also allows our mind to take a day off from the routine, to refresh itself and to find new enthusiasm for the next set of workouts.

Step 3: Weight Training

Increase the fat you burn through weight training

5

Several recent scientific studies have proven what most of the fitness community has known "intuitively" for years: Weight training (also known as strength training or resistance training) actually increases your fat burning ability during both exercise and rest. Think about it, the more active, lean muscle tissue you have, the more calories it takes to keep that tissue alive and functioning, regardless of the workloads. But some people fear that by doing resistance weight training as described here, they'll wind up looking like some beefcaked bodybuilder. Fortunately, that's not what happens. Adding that kind of substantial muscle mass is extremely difficult to do and requires a six-day per week, heavy weight training program in conjunction

The Key Weight Training Concepts

▶ Choose the right place to weight train.

▶ Choose the right equipment.

▶ Weight train twice a week.

▶ Do 10–15 repetitions of each exercise.

▶ Do three sets of each exercise.

▶ Work all your major muscle groups in every strength workout.

▶ Stretch between exercises and afterward.

with much higher amounts of food than are outlined in this program and much less aerobic training.

The main intention of the exercises in the Fat Burning Factors Program is to encourage your natural muscle tissue to burn as much fat as it possibly can, whether during exercise or at rest. However, there are other residual benefits. Depending on your previous level of exercise, you will also find yourself more toned in certain places (e.g. your buttocks, thighs, shoulders) as a result of strength training. By putting a half an inch on your deltoids (outer shoulders), you will appear to have proportionately lost an inch around your waist or hips. Women can often benefit from this toning secret more than men. The point is that most people will respond to this program by toning and firming up in all the right places, without adding any unwanted bulk. Most importantly, the Fat Burning Factors weight training program will help maximize the 24-hour fat-burning potential of all major muscle groups.

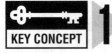 **1** *Choose the right place to weight train.*

As obvious as this concept may sound, choosing the right place to weight train is vital to your ability to stay motivated and to stick to the Fat Burning Factors Program. Many of us might be starting a training program for the first time, in which case the local health club or gym might seem a bit intimidating. After all, someone new to the concept of weight training might not be comfortable learning a new routine in full view of others. For these people, a home workout can work just as well as a full gym routine, provided they choose the right exercises *(Key Concept 2)* and can keep themselves motivated to train regularly. On the other hand, there are those of us who enjoy a health club or gym and who need the extra motivation provided by others who are involved in similar pursuits. The gym or health club is the perfect place to find other like-minded people. Also, there are usually more equipment choices at a larger health club or gym, most are staffed with knowledgeable trainers, and you'll even find that most fitness enthusiasts are all too happy to assist you in your learning process. Just be sure to choose a place that you know you'll want to go.

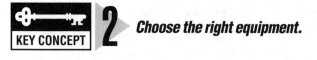 **KEY CONCEPT** **2** *Choose the right equipment.*

Walk into any health club or gym and you'll see anywhere from three to 25 ways to perform a "triceps extension" (the triceps is the muscle in the back of your arm that often sags and which many women accuse of being flabby). Although a triceps extension is one of the most basic weight training exercises, who can say which of those many choices is the best? Free weights or machines? Dumbbells, barbells or cables? Calisthenic, isometric or circuit? These are hard decisions to make, even if you understand the terminology and what each exercise accomplishes. The different equipment choices can be overwhelming and no one can say whether your selection of any one piece of equipment is absolutely better than choosing another. For this reason many veterans purposely change from one type of workout apparatus to another every few weeks. The best choice is what works best for you, so you enjoy it, see results and continue to do it. However, for whatever equipment or exercise you choose, there is a correct way to perform that specific exercise; and, if you do perform it correctly, you'll see the most measurable results. The most important thing is that you select a workout routine involving equipment that allows you to work each of the the major muscle groups through a full range of motion to a mild point of fatigue.

In view of the preceding statements, rather than pick one work-out routine for you and have you follow it blindly, we have chosen to offer a variety of popular workout routines—some for the home and some for the health club or gym—to allow you to decide which you prefer. As long as you stick to the one you select, you'll get the fat-burning benefits you seek. You'll find the routines at the end of this chapter with detailed instructions and photographs for each exercise.

KEY CONCEPT 3 ▶ *Weight train twice a week.*

Resistance training with weights, and even simple resistance training using your own body weight, constitutes a type of train-ing that is generally classified as anaerobic. This means that the muscles perform the exercises without using oxygen. Make no mistake, you can definitely get quite winded or out of breath doing anaerobic exercises, but this is a short-term effect. The out-of-breath feeling you experience lifting weights is not aer-obic, but the result of your body taking in more oxygen to "catch up" after a short burst of weight training exercise in order to fin-ish burning some of the carbohydrate you've only partially burned anaerobically. It's a bit complex, but the point is, when you do short sets of repetitions with an appropriate rest period in between, your body doesn't actually use much oxygen to perform these exercises. As a result, we can't burn much fat when we weight train—fat burning can only take place when there's lots of oxygen. Weight training burns mostly carbohydrate. You might ask why a fat-loss program would include anaerobic workouts, if the workouts themselves don't actually burn much fat. Our primary reason for doing this type of training is so we'll have more active muscle to burn off our stored fat 24 hours per day while we rest and while we are engaged in our aerobic activity.

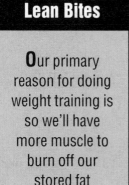

Lean Bites

Our primary reason for doing weight training is so we'll have more muscle to burn off our stored fat 24 hours a day.

Anaerobic workouts such as resistance training require a little longer recovery time between workouts. Whereas our muscles usually recover from and adapt to a medium effort aerobic workout (e.g., bicycling, climbing, walking, running, etc.) within 24 hours, it is better to allow between 48 and 72 hours rest between anaerobic strength training sessions. This is despite the fact that you may not feel like you need the rest. We get the most benefit from weight training only two times a week and allowing three or four days between sessions. Once per week is not quite enough to stimulate and retain the kind of muscle adaptations we want, and three or four times, while beneficial for some worldclass athletes, is not optimum for a program such as ours, which also includes four aerobic workouts each week. Your schedule might work best weight training Tuesday/Saturday or Monday/Thursday or Wednesday/Sunday, etc.

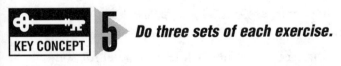

KEY CONCEPT 4 *Do 12-15 repetitions of each exercise.*

Each complete movement of a particular exercise is called a "repetition." Most anaerobic weight training workouts involve doing several "sets" of a certain number of repetitions. Over the years, several research studies have analyzed some of the different variables such as amount of weight and number of repetitions in order to determine what effect these variables have on the size and function of the muscle being trained. A general rule of thumb has emerged from these studies that says we should lift heavier weights for fewer repetitions to gain in size (bulk) and overall strength; and, we should lift lighter weights for a greater number of repetitions to build strength and endurance without as much increase in size.

Using this rule of thumb, and following the research, the Fat Burning Factors Program generally calls for 12 to 15 repetitions per set of each exercise to reach mild fatigue and to maximize the strength and endurance effect, without building bulkier muscles.

KEY CONCEPT 5 *Do three sets of each exercise.*

Some of the same studies that looked at the effects the amount of weight and number of repetitions had on muscle development also looked at the number of sets of each exercise required to generate a change within the muscle. These researchers discovered that major benefits come as a result of the first three sets of any exercise, but that after a few sets of each exercise, there is a dramatic drop in the incremental benefits of adding still more sets. In other words, the studies found that doing two sets of each exercise provides more stimulation for muscle change than doing just one set. And, doing three sets provides even greater stimulus than doing two. But, after three sets, the additional benefits from doing a fourth, fifth or sixth set are not significantly greater. Apparently, after three sets, almost all the stress that is needed to cause muscle adaptation has been applied. Applying any further stress (more sets) only marginally stimulates further change. In fact, some people think that doing more than three sets increases the risk of injury and is just not worth the effort or that doing more than three sets can interfere with your body's recovery for the next workout.

KEY CONCEPT **6** ***Work all of your major muscle groups in every strength workout.***

Many people who train regularly with weights choose to split their routines into three- or four-day "rotations." For example, some serious bodybuilders are particularly adamant about working their legs and abdominal muscles one day, chest and shoulders the next day, back and arms the third day and then resting on the fourth day before beginning the rotation all over again. They do this so they can overload a particular muscle group on one day and then allow that same muscle group three or four days of rest and recovery while they overload a different muscle group the next day. Of course, bodybuilders do many more sets for each body part than we will ever do. And, they also eat more than we ever will, since they are looking to "bulk up" and maximize every possible muscle growth opportunity. Their split rotations also provide a convenient excuse for them to have to go to the gym every day.

On the other hand, we in the Fat Burning Factors Program are looking to lose fat first while at the same time retaining lean muscle mass. We must balance our aerobic workouts with our strength training workouts—and fit all this into normal lives. We don't want our strength training to interfere with our fat-burning aerobic work. The compromise we make is that on the two days we set aside to strength train, we must work all body parts. The good news, as we learned in *Key Concept 5*, is that nearly 90% of the muscle gains possible will occur after the first three sets of any specific exercise. As a result, in a one hour-workout, we can accomplish almost as much muscle adaptation as we could over a three-day period of split workouts. This allows us four more days each week to do our fat-burning aerobic work and one day of complete rest.

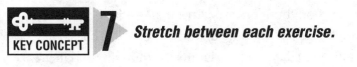 **KEY CONCEPT 7** *Stretch between each exercise.*

While strength is an important component of fitness and good health, it is equally important that our muscles retain their flexibility. An increase in strength does us little good if it causes us to become tight or inflexible. In order for our muscles to perform optimally and give us the greatest benefit in terms of fat-burning, they must be able to stretch and contract throughout their fullest range of motion. For this reason, a simple stretching program done between sets is an important part of your Fat Burning Factors anaerobic strength training routine. This stretching program takes advantage of the 60- to 90-second rest period between sets

Lean Bites

In order for our muscles to perform optimally and give us the greatest benefit in terms of fat-burning, they must be able to stretch and contract throughout their fullest range of motion.

and adds flexibility to your workout without adding any time.

FAT BURNING FACTORS™

THE WORKOUTS

The following workouts are intended as suggestions only. Before you undertake this or any diet or exercise program, be sure to consult with your physician.

FAT BURNING FACTORS™

HOME ROUTINE 1

No equipment is necessary, but you may need a towel, an armless chair and a post or a door.

1 ▶ ABDOMINAL CRUNCHES
For the muscles of the upper abdomen

2 ▶ BACK EXTENSIONS
For the muscles of the lower back and buttocks

3 ▶ REVERSE CRUNCHES
For the muscles of the lower abdomen

4 ▶ PUSH-UPS
For the muscles of the chest, shoulders, back of the arms and upper back

5 ▶ CHAIR DIPS
For the muscles of the chest, shoulders and back of the arms

6 ▶ TOWEL SQUATS
For the front and back of the upper thighs and buttocks

7 ▶ CALF RAISES
For the muscles of the back of the lower legs

1 ABDOMINAL CRUNCHES

Home
Routine 1

3 SETS

▶ *25-30 repetitions per set*

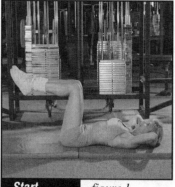

Start   *figure 1*

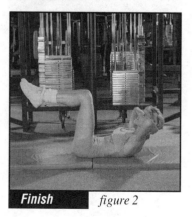

Finish   *figure 2*

Start by lying on the floor with your hands clasped loosely behind your head and your knees bent at a 90-degree angle *(figure 1)*. Slowly bring your head off the ground and squeeze or "crunch" your abdominal muscles tightly. Keep your neck relaxed—do all the work with your abdominal muscles *(figure 2)*. Do three sets of these abdominal crunches, up to 30 repetitions for each set with a short rest and some stretching in between sets. If you are able to perform more than 30 repetitions with the tightest contraction possible, carefully hold a weight behind your neck or across your chest to add more resistance.

2 BACK EXTENSIONS

Home
Routine 1

3 SETS PER SIDE

▶ *10 repetitions per set*

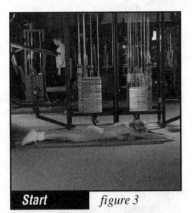

Start   *figure 3*

Finish   *figure 4*

Lying face down on the floor with your arms reaching out in front of you and your legs extended back *(figure 3)*, raise your left arm off the floor while simultaneously raising your right leg *(figure 4)*. Hold each approximately four to six inches off the floor for one second and then lower them. More advanced exercisers can hold for two or three seconds. Then do the same thing with your right arm and left leg. Alternate each side until you have completed 10 on each side.

3 REVERSE CRUNCHES

Home
Routine 1

3 SETS

▶ *15 repetitions per set*

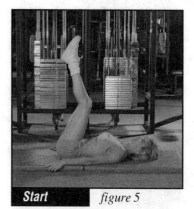

Start *figure 5*

Finish *figure 6*

Lie on your back on the ground, with your knees bent slightly and your ankles together (or feet crossed, if you prefer). Place your hands on the floor by your sides to stabilize yourself *(figure 5)*. As you exhale, curl your hips up toward the ceiling, using just your lower abdominal muscles. Lift your hips no more than about four inches *(figure 6)*. Make sure the middle of your back is on the ground at all times. Inhale as you return to the starting position.

4 *PUSH-UPS*

Home
Routine 1

3 SETS

▶*Each set to mild exhaustion*

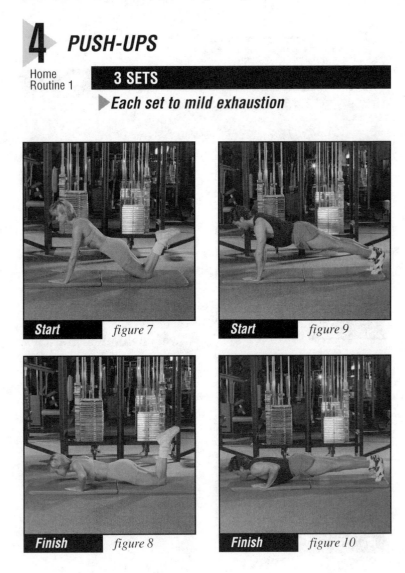

Start   *figure 7*

Start   *figure 9*

Finish   *figure 8*

Finish   *figure 10*

Beginners can do "half push-ups." Kneel on all fours with your knees shoulder-width apart and fingers pointing forward *(figure 7)*. Without allowing your back to sag, lower your chest to within an inch of the ground *(figure 8)* and then push back to the starting position. Keeping your abdominal muscles tightened as you perform the push-up will help keep your back from slouching. As you get stronger, you can do a full push-up where you support yourself with just your hands and feet *(figures 9 and 10)*.

5 CHAIR DIPS

Home
Routine 1

3 SETS

▶*Each set to exhaustion*

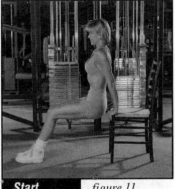

Start   *figure 11*

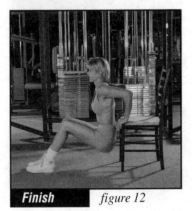

Finish   *figure 12*

Sit at the edge of a very stable armless chair and grasp the front edges of the chair with your hands. Place your feet on the ground with your knees bent at a 90-degree angle. Slide your buttocks off the chair to attain the starting position *(figure 11)*. Now, keeping your elbows in close to your sides, slowly lower your torso until your hands are just about at armpit level *(figure 12)*. When you reach the bottom of the movement, slowly press yourself back to the starting position. To increase the intensity, you can straighten one leg out as you dip down. Stronger participants can elevate both legs on another chair to increase resistance.

6 ▶ *TOWEL SQUATS*

Home
Routine 1

3 SETS (TOGETHER OR PER LEG)

▶ *15 repetitions per set*

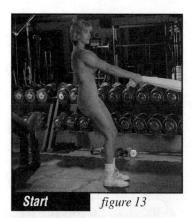

Start   *figure 13*

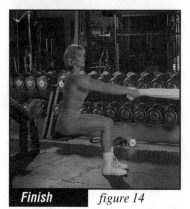

Finish   *figure 14*

Find a stable stationary post or open a door so that both doorknobs are visible. Wrap a towel around the post or one door knob, taking a stance a little less than at an arm's length away from it. Lean back slightly so the towel pulls on it *(figure 13)*. Keeping a straight back, slowly bend the knees lowering yourself until there is a 90-degree bend at your knees, inhaling as you descend *(figure 14)*. Now exhale as you slowly raise yourself back up to the starting position. If you are strong enough to do one leg at a time, do so alternating left then right, etc.

7 ▶ CALF RAISES

Home
Routine 1

3 SETS PER SIDE
▶ *20 repetitions per set*

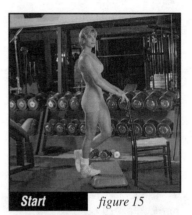

Start   *figure 15*

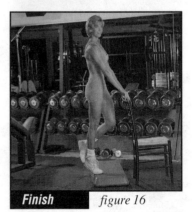

Finish   *figure 16*

Find a platform at least six inches off the ground. A bottom stair landing works well. Using a wall, a railing or a chair to help balance yourself, position one foot so that only the ball of the foot is in contact with the platform, with the remainder of the foot hanging off the side. Putting all your weight on that foot, slowly lower your foot so that your heel is below the level of the platform until you feel a slight stretch in your calf or Achilles tendon *(figure 15)*. Then slowly elevate yourself to a "tip-toe" position and hold it for one second *(figure 16)*. Do a full 20 repetitions and then switch feet and do 20 with the other.

FAT BURNING FACTORS™

► HOME ROUTINE 2

Minimal equipment purchase (less than $100). You'll need to purchase a flat bench and two matching dumbbells of a size or weight that allows you to do 10-15 repetitions of the following exercises:

1 ► **ABDOMINAL CRUNCHES**
For the muscles of the upper abdomen

2 ► **BACK EXTENSIONS**
For the muscles of the lower back and buttocks

3 ► **REVERSE CRUNCHES**
For the muscles of the lower abdomen

4 ► **PUSH-UPS**
For the muscles of the chest, shoulders, upper arms and upper back

5 ► **REAR DELTOID RAISE**
For the muscles of the shoulder and upper back

6 ► **DUMBBELL FLYES**
For the muscles of the chest and shoulders

7 ► **LATERAL RAISES**
For the muscles of the shoulders

8 ► **DUMBBELL CURLS**
For the muscles of the front of the arms

9 ► **SINGLE LAT ROWS**
For the muscles of the upper and middle back and front of the arm

10 **TRICEPS EXTENSIONS**
For the muscles of the back of the arm

11 **DUMBBELL LUNGES**
For the muscles in the upper thigh and the buttocks

1▶ ABDOMINAL CRUNCHES

Home
Routine 2

3 SETS

▶ *25-30 repetitions per set*

As described on page 91
(figures 1 and 2)

2▶ BACK EXTENSIONS

Home
Routine 2

3 SETS PER SIDE

▶ *15 repetitions per set*

As described on page 92
(figures 3 and 4)

3▶ REVERSE CRUNCHES

Home
Routine 2

3 SETS

▶ *15 repetitions per set*

As described on page 93
(figures 5 and 6)

4▶ PUSH-UPS

Home
Routine 2

3 SETS

▶ *Each set to mild exhaustion*

As described on pages 94-95
(figures 7 and 8 or figures 9 and 10)

5 *REAR DELTOID RAISES*

Home
Routine 2

3 SETS

▶ *12-15 repetitions per set*

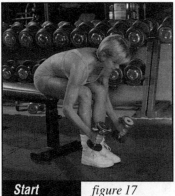

Start   *figure 17*

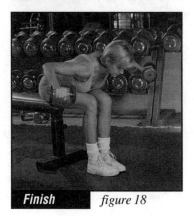

Finish   *figure 18*

Sit on the edge of your bench. Lean slightly forward, keeping your spine straight *(figure 17)*. With dumbbells in your hands, palms facing inward, slowly raise your arms out to the sides. Exhale as you complete this motion. A slight bend in the arms at the elbow is OK. Once your arms are raised to a level even with your back, squeeze your shoulder blades together *(figure 18)*, then slowly return your arms to the starting position as you inhale.

6 ▶ DUMBBELL FLYES

Home
Routine 2

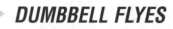

3 SETS

▶ *12-15 repetitions per set*

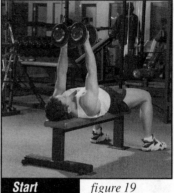

Start *figure 19*

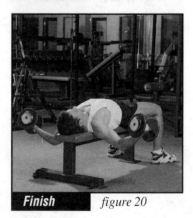

Finish *figure 20*

Grab a dumbbell in each hand and lie back on the bench, with your feet flat on the floor. Start with the dumbbells touching each other, your palms facing inward *(figure 19)*. With the arms still extended, bend slightly at your elbows and allow the dumbbells to move slowly out to the sides and down in an arc as you inhale *(figure 20)*. Using your chest muscles, return the dumbbells to the starting position by following the same arc back as you exhale.

7 ▶ *LATERAL RAISES*

Home
Routine 2

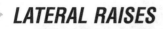

3 SETS

▶*12-15 repetitions per set*

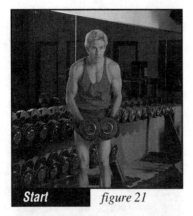

Start   *figure 21*

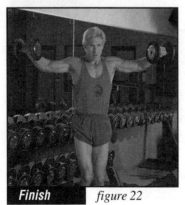

Finish   *figure 22*

Stand with your feet shoulder width apart, holding a dumbbell in each hand, palms facing inward *(figure 21)*. Simultaneously raise both dumbbells up and to the side just above shoulder level, maintaining a slight bend at the elbow *(figure 22)*. Exhale as you execute the move. Slowly lower dumbbells to the starting position as you inhale. To alter the point of stress on the shoulder muscles, you can vary this exercise a little by bending forward slightly at the hips.

8 DUMBBELL CURLS

Home
Routine 2

3 SETS

▶ *12-15 repetitions per set*

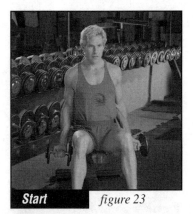

Start   *figure 23*

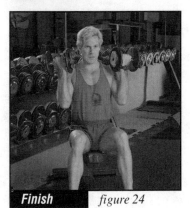

Finish   *figure 24*

Sit upright on the bench, holding a dumbbell in each hand, with your arms extended fully, palms facing forward and elbows close to your sides *(figure 23)*. Exhale as you slowly curl your arms up to your shoulders, keeping your elbows close to your waist *(figure 24)*. Don't use your back. Slowly lower the dumbbells back to the starting position, inhaling as you do.

9 SINGLE LAT ROWS

Home
Routine 2

3 SETS PER SIDE

▶ *12-15 repetitions per set*

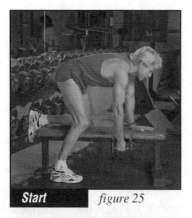

Start   *figure 25*

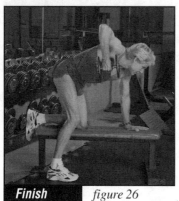

Finish   *figure 26*

Support yourself on the bench by placing your left hand and left knee on the bench and your right foot on the ground. Hold a dumbbell in your right hand allowing your arm to hang down from your shoulder *(figure 25)*. Keeping a flat back and your abdominals contracted, exhale and slowly draw your right elbow up, pulling your shoulder blades together as you lift, until the dumbbell is next to your ribs *(figure 26)*. Hold it there for a second and then inhale as you lower the weight slowly to the starting position. After doing 12-15 on the right side, switch positions and perform the next set on the left side, alternating sides until three sets are completed.

10 *TRICEPS EXTENSIONS*

Home
Routine 2

3 SETS PER SIDE

▶*12-15 repetitions per set*

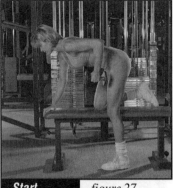

Start *figure 27*

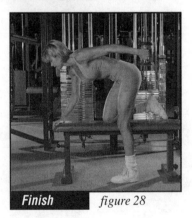

Finish *figure 28*

Support yourself on the bench by placing your right hand and right knee on the bench and your left foot on the ground. Hold a dumbbell in your left hand. Position the top of your left arm so that it is level with your back and your elbow is pressed against your side *(figure 27)*. Keeping a flat back and your abdominals contracted, exhale and slowly extend the left arm straight back, without moving your elbow from your side *(figure 28)*. Inhale as you relax and allow the dumbbell to hang at a 90-degree angle again. Do 12-15 on this side and then switch sides for the next set, alternating sides until three sets are completed.

11 *Dumbbell Lunges*

Home
Routine 2

3 SETS PER SIDE

▶*12-15 repetitions per set*

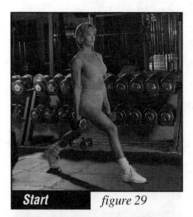

Start   *figure 29*

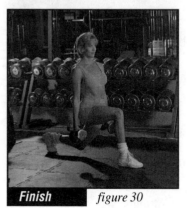

Finish   *figure 30*

Stand up straight, feet about 8 inches apart, holding a dumbbell in each hand, with your palms facing inward. Let the weights hang at your sides. Carefully take a large step forward with your right foot until your knee is almost over your foot *(figure 29)*. Now allow yourself to dip your left knee almost to the ground *(figure 30)* and then raise yourself back to the full extended position. Repeat this 12-15 times on this side and then reverse your stance and do a set on the other side, alternating sides until three sets are completed.

FAT BURNING FACTORS™

▶ GYM ROUTINE

This workout can be done at almost any health club or gym or in a well-equipped home gym. If you prefer, similar free weight exercises, like those mentioned earlier, can be substituted for the machine exercises described here.

1 ▶ ABDOMINAL CRUNCHES
For the muscles of the upper abdomen

2 ▶ BACK EXTENSIONS
For the muscles of the lower back and buttocks

3 ▶ REVERSE CRUNCHES
For the muscles of the lower abdomen

4 ▶ BENCH PRESS
For the muscles of the chest, shoulders and back of the arms

5 ▶ LAT PULL-DOWNS
For the muscles of the upper back and front of the arms

6 ▶ PEC FLYES
For the muscles of the chest and shoulders

7 ▶ LATERAL RAISES
For the muscles of the shoulders

8 ▶ BICEPS CURLS
For the muscles in the front of the arms

9 ▶ TRICEPS EXTENSIONS
For the muscles in the back of the arms

10 HAMSTRING CURLS
For the muscles in the back of the upper thighs

11 QUADRICEPS EXTENSIONS
For the muscles in the front of the thighs

FOR YOUR SAFETY

Whenever you use free weights, be sure to have a "spotter" nearby who can assist you in completing the exercise, should you encounter any difficulty. Also, be careful not to choose weights that are too heavy, especially when you are just starting out. Beginners should select weights that allow you to complete 15 repetitions without difficulty. Then, as you gain strength and confidence you can gradually (week by week) increase the amounts of weight until muscular fatigue makes it difficult to complete the 15th repetition.

ABDOMINAL CRUNCHES

Gym
Routine

3 SETS

▶*25-30 repetitions per set*

As described on page 91
(figures 1 and 2)

 BACK EXTENSIONS

Gym
Routine

3 SETS PER SIDE

▶*15 repetitions per set*

As described on page 92
(figures 3 and 4)

REVERSE CRUNCHES

Gym
Routine

3 SETS

▶*15 repetitions per set*

As described on page 93
(figures 5 and 6)

4 ▶ *BENCH PRESS*

Gym
Routine

3 SETS

▶*12-15 repetitions per set*

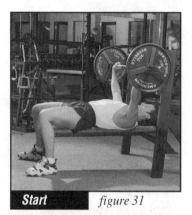

Start   *figure 31*

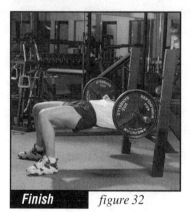

Finish   *figure 32*

Lie on the bench with your back flat on the bench and your feet flat on the ground. Grasp the bar with your hands spaced slightly more than shoulder width apart. Press the barbell off the rack and position it so that it is directly above your chest *(figure 31)*. Slowly lower the barbell to your chest *(figure 32)*, inhaling as you lower and then press it back to the position above your chest, exhaling as you press. Don't arch your back while performing this exercise.

5 ▶ LAT PULL-DOWNS

Gym
Routine

3 SETS

▶*12-15 repetitions per set*

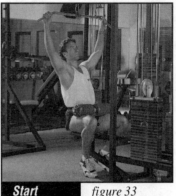

Start   *figure 33*

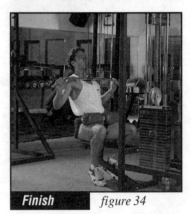

Finish   *figure 34*

Sit on the bench with a slight arch in your back and your legs under the support. Grab the bar with a wide overhand grip, preferably on the descending or bent parts of the bar *(figure 33)*. Maintaining a slight arch, pull the bar down until it just touches the top of your chest, exhaling as you pull down *(figure 34)*. Slowly allow the bar to return to the starting position as you inhale.

6 ▶ *PEC FLYES*

Gym
Routine

3 SETS

▶ *12-15 repetitions per set*

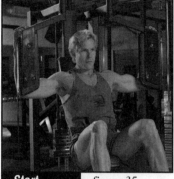

Start *figure 35*

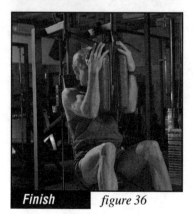

Finish *figure 36*

Seated at the pec deck machine, place your forearms on the arm pads so that there is a 90-degree bend at your elbows. Inhale and allow the pads to return to the starting position, which should produce a mild stretch in the pectoral muscles of your chest *(figure 35)*. As you exhale, slowly squeeze your arms together until the pads touch in front of you *(figure 36)*, pausing slightly when they do touch, then let the pads return to the starting position as you inhale.

7 ▶ *LATERAL RAISES*

Gym
Routine

3 SETS

▶*12-15 repetitions per set*

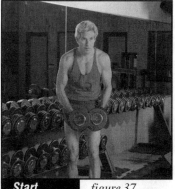

Start   *figure 37*

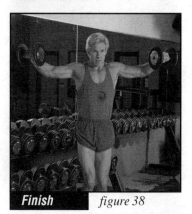

Finish   *figure 38*

Stand with your feet shoulder width apart, holding a dumbbell in each hand, palms facing inward *(figure 37)*. Simultaneously raise both dumbbells up and to the side just above shoulder level, maintaining a slight bend at the elbow *(figure 38)*. Exhale as you execute the move. Slowly lower the dumbbells to the starting position as you inhale. To alter the point of stress on the shoulder muscles, you can vary this exercise a little by bending forward slightly at the hips.

8 ▶ BICEPS CURLS

Gym
Routine

3 SETS

▶ *12-15 repetitions per set*

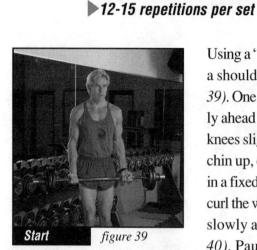

Start *figure 39*

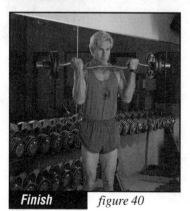

Finish *figure 40*

Using a "curling barbell," take a shoulder width grip *(figure 39)*. One foot should be slightly ahead of the other and both knees slightly bent. With your chin up, chest out and elbows in a fixed position at your side, curl the weight up to your chin slowly as you exhale *(figure 40)*. Pause for a second and then lower it back to the starting point as you inhale. Do not use your back to assist you with this movement.

9 *TRICEPS EXTENSIONS*

Gym
Routine

3 SETS

▶*12-15 repetitions per set*

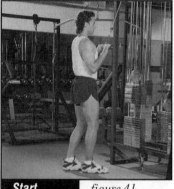

Start   *figure 41*

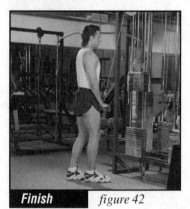

Finish   *figure 42*

Stand close to the overhead cable pulley and take an overhand grip on the bar. Your hands should be no further than 8 inches apart, and your knees slightly bent *(figure 41)*. Keeping your elbows in close to your sides, exhale as you press the bar down by extending your arms at the elbow *(figure 42)*. Slowly allow the bar to return to the starting position as you inhale.

10 HAMSTRING CURLS

Gym
Routine

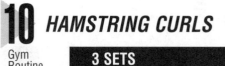

3 SETS

▶ *12-15 repetitions per set*

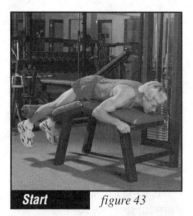

Start   *figure 43*

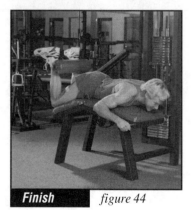

Finish   *figure 44*

Lie face down on a hamstring machine bench so that your knees extend just over the edge of the bench. Place your heels behind the pads and steady yourself with your hands by grasping the side of the bench, or handles if provided *(figure 43)*. Exhale as you slowly curl your heels toward your buttocks, making sure to keep your hips in contact with the bench *(figure 44)*. Pause and then slowly lower the weight back to the starting position as you inhale.

117

11 *QUADRICEPS EXTENSIONS*

Gym
Routine

3 SETS

▶*12-15 repetitions per set*

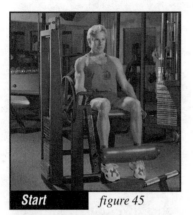

Start   *figure 45*

Finish   *figure 46*

Sit in the seat so that your knee is positioned directly over the edge of the seat and your back is against the back rest. The fronts of your ankles should be underneath the roller pads *(figure 45)*. Exhale as you extend your legs out straight in front of you *(figure 46)*. Pause momentarily before lowering the weight to the starting position as you inhale. You can do both legs at the same time or alternate one leg at a time.

FAT BURNING FACTORS™

STRETCHING ROUTINE

These stretches should be performed between weight training sets when possible and always at the end of both your strength training and your aerobic workout. With any stretch, take a few moments to ease into the stretch position and then, once there, hold it for 20-30 seconds while relaxing that muscle or muscle group.

1 **GROIN STRETCH**
For the muscles of the groin and inner thigh

2 **ACHILLES TENDON AND CALF STRETCH**
For the muscles of the back of the lower leg

3 **CHEST AND SHOULDER STRETCH**
For the muscles of the chest and shoulders

4 **BUTTOCKS STRETCH**
For the muscles of the buttocks and back of the upper leg

5 **HAMSTRING/QUAD STRETCH**
For the muscles of the front and back of the upper leg

1 ▶ *GROIN STRETCH*

RELAX AND HOLD POSITION

▶ *20-30 seconds*

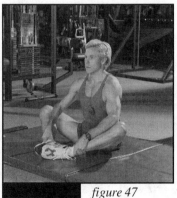

figure 47

Sit on the floor with your knees out to the sides and the bottoms of your feet touching each other. Pull your feet in as close to your groin as possible. Relax your legs and with your hands at your ankles, use your elbows to gently press your knees toward the floor until you feel a slight stretch *(figure 47)*. Hold that position for 20-30 seconds and then relax.

2 ACHILLES TENDON & CALF STRETCH

Stretching
Routine

RELAX AND HOLD POSITION

▶*20-30 seconds per leg*

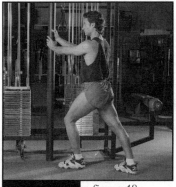

figure 48

Stand three to four feet away from a wall and lean into it, supporting yourself with your hands on the wall. Bend one leg at the knee and extend the other straight out behind you and away from the wall. Keep the extended foot flat on the floor while slowly moving your hips toward the wall and bending the extended leg slightly at the knee until you feel a stretch in your calf and/or Achilles tendon *(figure 48)*. Don't let your heel lift off the floor. Hold that position for 20-30 seconds and then repeat the stretch for the opposite leg.

3 CHEST & SHOULDER STRETCH

Stretching
Routine

RELAX AND HOLD POSITION

▶*20-30 seconds*

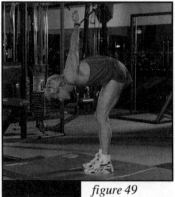

figure 49

Extend your arms behind you so that you can clasp your hands together. Roll your clasped hands down and around so that your thumbs are pointing toward the floor. Bend forward at the hips and allow your arms to come up over your back until you feel a stretch in your chest and shoulders *(figure 49)*. Hold it for 20-30 seconds. Depending on how far you lean forward, this is also an excellent stretch for the lower back and the back of the upper legs.

4 ▶ *BUTTOCKS STRETCH*

Stretching
Routine

RELAX AND HOLD POSITION

▶ *20-30 seconds per side*

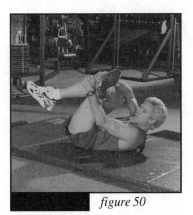

figure 50

Lie on your back and tuck your left knee behind your right ankle. Place your hands on your left shin—one over the right leg and one under as pictured—and pull your knee toward you. By pulling your knee in, you will begin to feel a stretch in your right buttocks (figure 50). Hold that position for 20-30 seconds and then reverse position to stretch the opposite buttocks.

5 ▷ *HAMSTRING/QUAD STRETCH*

Stretching
Routine

RELAX AND HOLD EACH POSITION

▷ *20-30 seconds per leg*

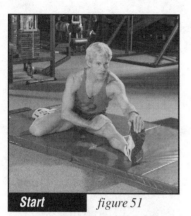

Start   *figure 51*

Finish   *figure 52*

Assume a "modified hurdlers position" so that your left leg is extended out in front of you and your right leg is bent at the knee. To stretch your left hamstring, lower yourself toward your knee, trying to touch your chest to your knee, while maintaining a straight back. As soon as you begin to feel the hamstring muscles in the back of the thigh stretch, hold that position for 20-30 seconds *(figure 51)*. Then, to stretch the quadriceps of the opposite leg, lean backwards, supporting yourself with your arms, until you feel a slight stretch and hold that position *(figure 52)*. Reverse the hurdlers position to stretch alternate legs.

Real Meals

How to select and prepare healthy, tasty, satisfying foods

It isn't always easy to buy and prepare healthy, tasty foods, especially with today's fast-paced lifestyle. However, whenever possible, shop for *fresh* foods because they are always best. If you know that there won't be time to cook a fresh-food meal, you may opt for plain, frozen foods, but avoid those with added butter, cheese, cream, margarine and sauces.

The way food is prepared can determine whether your body will get all the recommended vitamins, minerals, protein, fat and carbohydrates. Although all your needed nutrients might be in your food, if the food is not cooked properly, the nutrients might not have their intended effect. Below are some general guidelines for cooking any healthy meal:

General Guidelines for Cooking any Healthy Meal:

1. Cut down on your use of oils, butter and margarines. Use non-stick cooking sprays. When you can't avoid using oil, choose canola or olive oil. Try Butter Buds or Molly McButter on vegetables. When you must use butter or margarine, choose soft-tub margarine.

2. Substitute non-fat milk for low-fat or whole milk.

3. Substitute plain, non-fat yogurt for mayonnaise or sour cream.

4. Use non-fat milk or evaporated, non-fat milk thickened with a small amount of flour or corn starch instead of cream in sauces and gravies.

5. Use fresh herbs, spices and vinegars to add zest and flavor without adding fat.

6. Use vegetable purée as a healthy base for creamy soups.

7. Use non-fat or low-fat cottage cheese or non-fat cheese, instead of regular cheese.

8. Use Egg Beaters or just egg whites instead of whole eggs.

9. Steam, bake or broil (in little or no oil) instead of deep-frying in oil. If you stir-fry, use water or tamari instead of oil.

10. Stick to low-oil, low-fat or non-fat sauces and dressings.

11. Keep meat portions at any one meal under five ounces. Better yet, use meat as a flavoring for another dish (e.g., pasta, rice, salads, etc.) rather than as a main course.

12. Remove skin and trim any visible fat from all poultry and meats.

13. Substitute lean ground turkey for ground beef. Look for packages listing 7% fat or less.

14. Use dried beans and dried peas in place of meat.

EATING OUT

There may be occasions when you won't have the time or the desire to cook a slow, healthy meal, and a fast-food restaurant is all that is available. In fact, a Gallup poll found that 37% of all Americans eat fast food eight or more times per month. Below are some general fast food tips:

Fast-Food, Low-Fat Hints:

1. With fast food, always beware of the skin on chicken, high fat sauces and added cheese.

2. Substitute mustard and/or ketchup for mayonnaise or tartar sauce on your sandwich or burger.

3. Try a salad and baked potato, but avoid adding butter, sour cream and bacon bits. Ask for low-fat dressing on the side.

4. Choose thin-crusted pizza instead of the deep-dish varieties. Go easy on the cheese and try low-fat, low calorie toppings like lean ham, mushrooms, onions, peppers, pineapple, shrimp and tomatoes.

5. Avoid fat-laden side dishes like potato and macaroni salads, biscuits and cornbread and most cole slaws. Instead, opt for baked potato, corn on the cob, rice, vegetables or a salad.

6. Avoid chicken wings or any other fried or battered appetizers served with heavy dipping sauces.

Low-Fat Fast Food Choices:

- Taco Bell's Border Light soft taco or bean burrito
- El Pollo Loco's chicken breast or chicken taco
- Boston Chicken's ¼ chicken, white meat or chicken breast sandwich
- Jack In The Box's chicken teriyaki bowl
- Arby's roast turkey deluxe sandwich
- Carl's Jr.'s grilled barbecue chicken sandwich
- McDonald's McGrilled chicken classic
- Subway's veggie and cheese or ham and cheese sandwiches
- Wendy's grilled chicken sandwich
▶ Domino's hand-tossed veggie pizza
- Little Caesar's cheese pizza
▶ Pizza Hut's hand-tossed ham pizza
- Thin 'N Crispy's hand-tossed veggie lover's pizza

▶ *We all dine in restaurants from time to time, but the choices are often overwhelming. The tips that follow will help insure that we continue in the fat-burning mode when we dine out.*

Restaurant Strategies:

1. Avoid filling up on bread or chips before your main course arrives. If you need an appetizer before your main course, order a salad (with low-fat dressing on the side and no meat or cheese), a raw or steamed vegetable dish or a clear, broth-based soup.

2. Drink water or herbal or decaffeinated iced tea before or after your meal. Limit your alcohol intake to one or fewer drinks per day.

3. Stay away from entrees with heavy cream- or oil-based sauces.

4. Stick to foods that are steamed, baked, broiled, grilled or sautéed in broth or wine, not oil or butter.

5. Don't feel obliged to finish everything. Most restaurants serve far more than you'd normally serve yourself at home. Ask for a take-out box and save what you don't eat for another meal.

6. Improvise. Most restaurants will gladly modify any dish to accommodate your needs. If nothing on the menu appeals to you, ask for a large plate of steamed vegetables; a pasta with a marinara sauce; or a broiled or grilled fish or chicken dish without the sauce.

7. For dessert, order fresh fruit, fruit ices or non-fat sherbet.

SAMPLE MEALS AND SNACKS

Whether you eat at home or dine out, the following meal and snack suggestions will give you some idea of the range of foods that fit into the Fat Burning Factors Program. While these meals vary somewhat in their relative mix of carbohydrate, protein and fat, they all fall well within an acceptable range, provided you vary the combinations of breakfasts, lunches, dinners and snacks. To account for your own personal caloric needs, vary the portion sizes or the number of snacks between meals accordingly. Remember, these represent just a few of the countless options available that make eating healthy both easy and satisfying. Use these suggestions as a starting point for introducing healthy meal ideas of your own.

Sample Healthy Meals

▶ *BREAKFASTS*

If you are so inclined, cup of coffee or tea is fine with any breakfast. But, try to use non-fat, or if you must, low-fat milk instead of cream; sugar is OK. Any type of fruit juice or water is also OK.

▶ French toast with fruit and syrup (very little butter)

▶ Hot oatmeal with fruit and non-fat yogurt

▶ Omelet made with any combination of spinach, tomatoes, mushrooms, herbs and salsa, with toast, muffin or bagel. Use one yolk and two or three egg whites.

▶ Potato-and-vegetable hash with chicken or tofu flavoring

▶ Low-fat cottage cheese with fruit

▶ Fruit bowl topped with yogurt

▶ Huevos rancheros (Mexican omelet with salsa)

▶ Whole-wheat or oatmeal-banana pancakes with fruit syrup and tofu breakfast links

▶ Bowl of Müeslix or low-fat granola, with non-fat milk and fruit

▶ Bagel with lox and "lite" or non-fat cream cheese

▶ Whole-wheat waffle with strawberries and maple syrup

▶ Whole-wheat toast with a fruit milkshake (skim milk)

▶ Melba toast with a thin layer of low-fat, natural peanut butter

Sample Healthy Meals

▶ *LUNCHES*

Try any of the following drinks with your lunch: tea, mineral water, non-fat milk, non-alcoholic beer or wine, sparkling water or juice.

▶ Tuna salad sandwich with seven-grain bread and fruit ("lite" mayonnaise and tuna packed in water)

▶ Chicken salad sandwich on whole wheat, rye, pumpernickel or multi-grain bread with chicken soup

▶ Broiled turkey or veggie burger on whole wheat bun with ketchup or mustard served with fruit

▶ Sliced turkey sandwich on whole-wheat or multi-grain bread with "lite" cheese and grated carrots (light on the mayonnaise)

▶ Any variable mixture of steamed vegetables with rice, baked potato or pita bread

▶ Vegetable salad with small portions of turkey or chicken with vinaigrette dressing

▶ Baked or charbroiled fish with mashed potatoes

▶ Pasta with clam sauce or low-oil marinara sauce

▶ Scrambled tofu served with bread and fruit

▶ Vegetarian burrito

Sample Healthy Meals

DINNERS

Have any of the following drinks with your dinner: sparkling, mineral or spring water, wine or beer, caffeine-free tea, caffeine-free soft drink, non-alcoholic beer or wine.

▶ Broiled or baked salmon with steamed vegetables

▶ Chicken chow mein with rice

▶ Baked potatoes with sauce of mushrooms sautéed in tamari, served with steamed vegetables

▶ Vegetable salad with chicken or turkey strips and low-oil or "lite" salad dressing

▶ Green peppers stuffed with ground turkey (or extra lean ground beef) and brown rice

▶ Turkey with vegetables and sweet potato (no gravy)

▶ Stir-fried chicken (or tofu) with vegetables and ginger

▶ Chicken marinara with vegetables and salad

▶ Vegetarian chili with whole-wheat bread

▶ Soup and salad with whole-wheat bread

▶ Pasta cooked with a little olive oil, garlic, herbs, black pepper and Parmesan cheese, served with steamed vegetables

▶ Stir-fried seafood with fresh vegetables and brown rice

Sample Healthy Meals

DESSERTS

Have a tasty, low-fat dessert and enjoy it without feeling guilty.

- Angel food cake topped with fresh fruit and non-fat whipped topping
- Sorbet or fruit ice in center of cantaloupe
- Frozen fruit bars
- Fresh fruit with non-fat yogurt
- Drizzle non-fat lemon yogurt over sugar-free flavored gelatin
- Fresh, natural applesauce with granola
- Baked apples with cinnamon, ginger, diet soda and rum extract
- ▶ Fresh apple, orange, banana and canned pineapple in its own juice folded into instant, sugar-free vanilla pudding mix
- ▶ Sugar-free Jell-O with plain fat-free yogurt and fresh blueberries, strawberries and raspberries
- Baked stuffed pears with raisins, apple juice, fat-free yogurt, lemon juice and nutmeg
- ▶ Bread pudding made with egg substitute, skimmed milk, evaporated milk, vanilla, bread crumbs, raisins, apple slices and nutmeg

Sample Healthy Meals

SNACKS

Portion control is critical to healthful snacking. Avoid eating directly from any bulk package

- Air-popped popcorn (almost any amount)
- Half a bagel with low-fat spread
- Glass of non-alcoholic beer or wine
- One portion of any type of fresh fruit
- ▶ Glass of fruit or vegetable juice (any type)
- ▶ Pint of non-fat or "lite" yogurt
- ▶ Glass of non-fat milk
- Two rice cakes
- Two pieces of dried fruit
- ▶ Handful of pretzels
- ▶ Whole-grain bread or crackers
- Cup-A-Soup
- ▶ Bowl of whole-grain cereal with non-fat milk
- Handful of celery and/or carrot sticks
- Unsalted saltine or Ry-Krisp (unseasoned) crackers
- Four vanilla wafers, gingersnaps or animal crackers
- Two graham crackers or fig bars

FAT BITES

These are the tempting snack foods you should learn to avoid. If you indulge in any of these snack "fat bites," you'll need to do miles of extra credit aerobic exercise. If you absolutely have to have some, moderation is the key.

- Potato/tortilla chips with or without dip (e.g. guacamole or sour cream and onions)
- Dry-roasted or chocolate-covered nuts
- Candy bars (especially those with nuts), M&Ms and chocolate in general
- Pepperoni or sausage pizza
- Doughnuts, croissants and other pastries
- Ice cream
- French fries
- Cookies
- Puddings made with whole milk
- Meatballs
- Hamburgers and hotdogs
- Milkshakes
▶ Beer and other alcoholic drinks
▶ Nachos with melted cheese
- Fried anything

References

The research behind the Fat Burning Factors Lean Lifestyle Program

The Fat Burning Factors Lean Lifestyle Program is not merely the opinion of the authors. Rather, it is the conclusion of a careful review of literally thousands of research studies in the areas of weight loss, exercise physiology, biochemistry, medicine and nutrition. The following are a small sampling of the many reference papers, articles and other independent studies supporting the statements and recommendations contained in the Fat Burning Factors Program:

We can drastically reduce our likelihood of developing many different types of cancer simply by altering what we eat.
Newberne, P.M. and Conner, M.W. "Dietary modifiers of cancer." *Progress in Clinical and Biological Research* 1988; 259:105-129

Overweight men can reduce their risk of dying from cancer by losing body fat.
Wilcosky, T., Hyde, J., Anderson, J.J., Bangdiwala, S. and Duncan, B. "Obesity and mortality in the Lipid Research Clinics Program Follow-up Study." *Journal of Clinical Epidemiology* 1990; 43(8):743-52

As we gain more weight, our risk of dying from any and all types of diseases increases.
Lee, I-M. and Paffenbarger, R.S. "Change in body weight and longevity." *American Medical Association Journal* 1992; 268:2045-2049

There is strong evidence that many environmental toxins can accumulate in fat tissue.
Linder, R.E., Edgerton, T.R., Svendsgaard, D.J. and Moseman, R.F. "Long-term accumulation of hexachlorobenzene in adipose tissue of parent and filial rats." *Toxicology Letters* 1983 Feb; 15(2-3):237-43

Dragnev, K.H., Beebe, L.E., Jones, C.R., Fox, S.D., Thomas, P.E., Nims, R.W. and Lubet, R.A. "Subchronic dietary exposure to Aroclor 1254 in rats: accumulation of PCBs in liver, blood, and adipose tissue and its relationship to induction of various hepatic drug-metabolizing enzymes." *Toxicology and Applied Pharmacology* 1994 Mar; 125(1):111-22

Obesity can be a major cause of low back pain.
Deyo, R.A. and Bass, J.E. "Lifestyle and low-back pain. The influence of smoking and obesity." *Spine* 1989 May; 14(5):501-6

Many people who otherwise might have adult onset diabetes can avoid developing the condition if they lose body fat.
Long, S.D., O'Brien. K., MacDonald, K.G. Jr., Leggett-Frazier, N., Swanson, M.S., Pories, W.J. and Caro, J.F. "Weight loss in severely obese subjects prevents the pro-

gression of impaired glucose tolerance to Type II diabetes. A longitudinal interventional study." *Diabetes Care* 1994 May; 17(5):372-5

Overweight people are far more likely to develop adult onset diabetes than those who are leaner.
Maegawa, H., Kashiwagi, A. and Shigeta, Y. "Obesity as a risk factor for developing non-insulin dependent diabetes mellitus—obesity and insulin resistance." *Nippon Naibunpi Gakkai Zasshi* 1995 Mar 20; 71(2):97-104

Obese people often have lower self-esteem, personality distortions and lower self-satisfaction.
Stein, R.F. "Comparison of self-concept of non-obese and obese university junior female nursing students." *Adolescence* 1987; 22(85):77-90

Lean Body Mass can be used to determine the ideal calorie consumption in both men and women.
Webb, P. "Energy expenditure and fat-free mass in men and women." *American Journal of Clinical Nutrition* 1981; 34:1816-1826

Several short training sessions can be as effective as one longer session.
DeBusk, R.F., Stenestrand, U., Sheehan, M. and Haskell, W.L. "Training effects of long versus short bouts of exercise in healthy subjects." *American Journal of Cardiology* 1990; 65:1010-1013

The more intense the exercise, the more energy you expend, including more fat.
Bielinski, R., Schutz, Y. and Jequier, E. "Energy metabolism during the postexercise recovery in man." *American Journal of Clinical Nutrition* 1985 Jul; 42(1):69-82

A regular frequent exercise program can train your body to burn more calories (and hence more fat) each time you work out.
Martin, W.H., Dalsky, G.P., Hurley, B.F., et al. "Effect of endurance training on plasma free fatty acid turnover and oxidation during exercise." *American Journal of Physiology* 1993; 265:E708-E714

Aerobic exercise teaches the body to burn more fat at rest.
Berg, K.E. "Comparison of energy expenditure in men and women at rest and during exercise recovery." *Journal of Sports Medicine and Physical Fitness* 1991 Sep; 31(3):351-6

Four or five aerobic workouts per week provide optimum benefits, but the absolute minimum for anyone looking for fitness gains should be three times per week.
Gettman, L.R., Pollock, M.L., Durstine, J.L., Ward, A., Ayres, J. and Linnerud, A.C. "Physiological regarding enhancement of aerobic capacity." *Research Quarterly* 1977; 48:583-591

Wenger, H.A. and Bell, G.J. "The interactions of intensity, frequency and duration of exercise training in altering cardio-respiratory fitness." *Sports Medicine* 1986; 3:346-356

Training several times a week trains the body to burn more calories during every workout.
Moffatt, R.J., Stamford, B.A. and Neill, R.D. "Placement of tri-weekly training sessions: importance responses of men to 1-, 3-, and 5-day-per-week training programs." *Research Quarterly* 1976; 47:638-646

Strength training can result in substantial losses in body fat, while it simultaneously increases your lean muscle mass.
Treuth, M.S., Ryan, A.S., Pratley, R.E., et al. "Effects of strength training on total and regional body composition in older." *Journal of Applied Physiology* 1994; 77 (2):614-620

Atha, J. "Strengthening muscle." *Exercise and Sport Science Review* 1981; 9:1-73

MacDougal, J.D. "Morphological changes in human skeletal muscle following strength training and immobilization." *Human Muscle Power* 1986. Jones, N.L., McArtney, N. and McComas, A.J. Eds. Human Kinetics Publishers. Champaign, IL

Clark, H.H. "Development of muscular strength and endurance." *Physical Fitness Research Digest President's Council on Physical Fitness and Sports*. Washington, D.C., U.S. Government Printing Office, Jan.

Sample Workout Diary
Use the blank form on the following page to make copies.

▶ ON AEROBIC ACTIVITY DAYS

FAT BURNING FACTORS™   DATE _12-3-95_

TRAINING LOG

WEIGHT _137_   MOST RECENT BODY FAT% _26_

▶ AEROBIC ACTIVITY _WALKING_

CALORIES BURNED _____ (or) _3.2_ MILES x 100 = _320_ CALORIES

TIME SPENT _:52_   WORKING HEART RATE _130_

▶ ON STRENGTH TRAINING DAYS

FAT BURNING FACTORS™   DATE _12-4-95_

TRAINING LOG

WEIGHT _137_   MOST RECENT BODY FAT% _26_

▶ AEROBIC ACTIVITY _____

CALORIES BURNED _____ (or) ____ MILES x 100 = _____ CALORIES

TIME SPENT _____   WORKING HEART RATE _____

▶ STRENGTH TRAINING

EXERCISE	SET 1 WEIGHT/REPS	SET 2 WEIGHT/REPS	SET 3 WEIGHT/REPS
AB CRUNCH	25	30	25
REV. CRUNCH	10	12	10
BACK EXT.	15	15	15
BENCH PRESS	90 11	90 12	90 10
	60 12	6	

FAT BURNING FACTORS™ DATE _____

► *TRAINING LOG*

WEIGHT_____ MOST RECENT BODY FAT% _____

► *AEROBIC ACTIVITY* _____

CALORIES BURNED _____ (or) _____ MILES x 100 = _____ CALORIES

TIME SPENT _____ WORKING HEART RATE _____

► *STRENGTH TRAINING*

EXERCISE	SET 1 WEIGHT/REPS	SET 2 WEIGHT/REPS	SET 3 WEIGHT/REPS